Older People and Nursing:
Issues of Living in a Care Home

IF 3/2012

*This book is dedicated
to the older people
with whom we work
and have worked.*

Older People and Nursing:
Issues of Living in a Care Home

Edited by

Pauline Ford
MA(Gerontology), RGN, DHMS, CMS

and

Hazel Heath
MSc Advanced Clinical Practice (Care of the Elderly),
BA(Hons), DipN(Lond), CertEd,
FETC, ITEC, RGN, RCNT, RNT

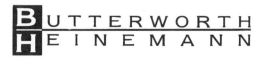

BUTTERWORTH
HEINEMANN

Butterworth-Heinemann
Linacre House, Jordan Hill, Oxford OX2 8DP
A division of Reed Educational & Professional Publishing Ltd

ℛ A member of the Reed Elsevier plc group

OXFORD   BOSTON   JOHANNESBURG
MELBOURNE   NEW DELHI   SINGAPORE

First published 1996

British Library Cataloguing in Publication Data
A catalogue record for this book is available from
the British Library

ISBN 0 7506 2438 8

Library of Congress Cataloguing in Publication Data
A catalogue record for this book is available from
the Library of Congress

Typesetting by David Gregson Associates, Beccles, Suffolk
Printed in Great Britain by Clays, St Ives plc

Contents

Foreword

Today, older people are the main consumers of nursing care and social services. Many older people can expect to enjoy a healthy old age, but the proportion of very old people who are frail and need care in a care home will increase as we move towards the end of the century. Today, older people who need to be cared for in a home, their relatives and carers face many dilemmas and anxieties.

The needs of older people are increasingly balanced against the need to contain costs and achieve greater efficiency in the provision of care. For too long, there has been a lack of clarity about who is responsible for the funding and provision of continuing care. Now at last, the continuing care of older people is a matter for wider debate and pressing concern for the Government and our health service.

The debate about continuing care has highlighted other issues surrounding the health care of older people. The move to the provision of nursing home care in the private sector, and the fact that people cared for in private nursing homes have had to pay for their nursing care as well as their accommodation in a way that no-one else who receives care through the NHS has to, is an important example. There is also a long standing problem of people who have been wrongly placed in residential homes when they need nursing care, and placed in nursing homes when they do not. Thus, finding cost effective and flexible solutions to the difficulties surrounding the care of frail older people is an urgent challenge for nurses, health service management, the Government, and other health care professionals alike.

There is no other area of health or medical care where the nurse's skills are more pre-eminent than in the care of older people. When the nursing care is of high quality, the older person receives support not just to recover from an acute episode of illness, but to reshape their lives, to recover and even improve their mobility. Nursing care enables many to face the future with confidence and enjoyment. At the same time, so many older people have multiple health care needs that can only be met by skilled and experienced nursing.

Skilled nursing care has also been proved time and again to be cost effective. Nurses are able to increase the choice and the volume of care available to their patients at a time when older people's choices appear to be diminishing. More people who are cared for by registered nurses get better more quickly. Many more are rehabilitated. They live longer and more comfortably. Furthermore, over the longer term, nursing care costs less.

If nurses who care for older people are to maintain the very highest standards of care, and continue to find flexible solutions to long term problems, nursing practice needs to be replenished and updated with new ideas and information on all aspects of the care of older people and the environment in which they are cared for. Increasingly, if nurses are to speak up for older people, they need to understand the national frame-work for care of which they are part, as well strengthening their clinical skills. Nurses need to know what is valuable about nursing care, and what older people value in nursing.

This book comprehensively examines these challenges. It is a valuable resource for all nurses who care for one of our most vulnerable patient groups.

Christine Hancock
General Secretary, Royal
College of Nursing

Contributors

Mary T. Clay MSc Advanced Clinical Practice (Care of the Elderly), RGN, RM
Matron, Moorlands Nursing Home, Lightwater, Surrey

Stuart J. Darby MBE, BA(Hons), RGN, RMN, RHV, DPSN
Formerly Head of Community Nursing Development Team, Camden and Islington Community Health Services NHS Trust; Chair of RCN Focus on Older People, Nursing and Mental Health

Pauline Ford MA (Gerontology), RGN, DHMS, CMS
Adviser on Nursing and Older People, Royal College of Nursing, London

Steve Goodwin RMN
National Co-ordinator of the Dark Horse Venture

Hazel Heath MSc Advanced Clinical Practice (Care of the Elderly), BA(Hons), DipN(Lond), Cert Ed, FETC, ITEC, RGN, RCNT, RNT
Independent Consultant, Lecturer and Writer, Chair of the RCN Association for the Care of Elderly People (ACE)

Glenda Hunter RGN, Cert (Gerontology), Dip (Gerontology)
Care Team Manager, Brownswood Nursing Home, London

Andrée Christine LeMay RGN, BSc(Hons), PhD, PGCEA
Principal Lecturer in Nursing, Department of Health Studies, Brunel University College, Isleworth

Jim Marr MA (Gerontology), BA (Educational Studies), DipCNE, RGN, RMN, RCNT, RNT
Consultant Nurse, Ashley Nursing Homes, Edinburgh; Vice Chair of RCN Focus on Older People, Nursing and Mental Health

Abigail Masterson MN, BSc, RGN, PGCEA
Lecturer in Primary Care Nursing, University of Bristol, Department of Social Medicine

Liz Matthew MA (Gerontology), RMN, RN, CPN Cert.
Directorate Manager, Mental Health Services (Older People), Community and Priority Services NHS Trust, Tameside General Hospital, Ashton-under-Lyne; Honorary Treasurer of RCN Focus on Older People, Nursing and Mental Health

Brendan McCormack BSc(Hons) Nursing, DPSN, PGCEA, RNT, RGN, RMN
Fellow/Programme Manager, National Institute for Nursing, and Oxfordshire Community Health NHS Trust; Co-opted Member of RCN Association for the Care of Elderly People (ACE)

Hilary Oliver RGN, FETC
Continence Adviser, Nurse Manager, Specialist Services, Bradford Community NHS Trust, Bradford, West Yorkshire

Helen Peace RGN
Senior Nurse, Elderly Services Directorate, The Ipswich Hospital NHS Trust, Ipswich, Suffolk

Lynne Phair BSc(Hons), RGN, RMN, DPNS
Team Leader, Mental Health Services for Older People, Eastbourne and County Healthcare NHS Trust, Hailsham, East Sussex; Honorary Treasurer of RCN Association for the Care of Elderly People (ACE)

Irene Schofield MSc, RGN, RNT, CertEd, Cert (Gerontology), Oncology Nursing Cert.
Lecturer in care of the older adult, City University, St Bartholomew School of Nursing and Midwifery

Maria Scurfield RMN, DPSN, BSc(Hons) Nursing Science
Clinical Nurse Manager, Priority Healthcare Wearside, Tyne and Wear; Honorary Secretary of RCN Focus on Older People and Nursing and Mental Health

Jane Slack RGN
Outreach Nurse, Weston Area Health Trust, Weston-super-Mare, North Somerset

Introduction

The editors believe that, as unique individuals, older people have their own life experiences, wisdom, values, interests, abilities, needs, and life tasks to perform. Each person also has a unique contribution to make to society, which does not cease on the basis of increasing age or infirmity, or the need for health and social care. Older age therefore should not be viewed as synonymous with decline, disability or ill-health but as a time with opportunities for new learning, health, happiness, fulfilment and growth.

Individuals age in different ways and react differently to the ageing experience. The only sure thing about older people is that they have lived longer than those who are younger. The life experiences accumulated during the past century encompass some of the most profound changes encountered by any one group of people: life-threatening deprivation, fundamental changes in social structure, unboundaried geographical mobility encompassing travel to other planets, and technological change. At the forefront of these changes have been older people. Their life events have given them a richness of perspective and sets of values without which society would be impoverished.

This book is for nurses working in care settings where older people live. While some of this care takes places within NHS settings, it is the private and voluntary sectors which predominate. Some older people will have their care needs met in their own homes, and the editors believe that the fundamental principles and values expressed in this book are equally applicable, whatever the setting for care.

Nurses will increasingly find themselves working in new environments and in new ways. Their ability to work creatively and innovatively with older people indicates that their value and skill will be scrutinised, and ultimately recognised.

Registered nurses working with older people can personally use this book to enhance their knowledge. Care workers may also find aspects of this book helpful. Ultimately we hope that the book will act not only as a resource, but also as a stimulus for questioning reflective practice.

The book is composed of a selection of papers reflecting key issues for nursing and older people. It is not intended to be an all-encompassing reference. Rather, it aims to draw together some of the priority issues in the view of the editors. The book has been compiled to reflect the individuality of the contributors, all of whom express their unique and specific contribution to working with older people.

The book is divided into three sections. The first, entitled National Frameworks and Values, consists of four chapters covering the key influencing factors in the provision of continuous care for older people today. The second section, entitled Quality of Life Matters, explores the key aspects that clearly have a direct impact on how an older person, and the staff, experience life in a setting providing continuous care. This section seeks to emphasise the interrelationship between staff values and quality of life for older people. The third section deals with selected Clinical Matters which the editors consider to be some of the current priorities.

The reader will be aware of the health and social policy influences in relation to the provision of care services. Increasingly opportunities now exist for older people to receive services from nurses in a variety of settings. Consequently this book is likely to be of interest to any nurse who works with older people on a continuing basis. For example, nurses may work within health centres, the community, housing associations, care homes, commissioning agencies and NHS units. These nurses will have a variety of employers, terms and conditions of service, and working experiences. The common factor to all will be a desire to continually strive towards a service provision that older people both need and want.

This book is written at a time of unprecedented change, and events may overtake its publication. At the time of writing, there is no indication of a lessening of such change. Accordingly there will continue to be a need for nurses to work creatively and responsively to ensure that older people continue to have the right to access the skills of nursing whenever they so choose.

Both the older people who live in continuing care settings, and the nurses who work with them, have traditionally been undervalued. Underinvestment and, more recently, active withdrawal has been widespread. Historically in the NHS, nurses in continuing care have worked in the worst accommodation, with the least facilities and equipment of all care settings, and there has been a history of educational neglect. Despite this some of the most well-known good practice within the NHS has taken place within continuing care settings.

For nurses who work in care homes there are specific challenges. These nurses often work in professional isolation, either in a small home or alone on duty as the only RGN on the shift. This means that some of the professional support which their colleagues in the statutory sector can take for granted, like mentorship, peer review and supervision, will be more challenging to achieve. Nurses working in care homes may have far greater difficulty in accessing colleges of education, conferences, study leave and peer support. This book aims to redress the balance.

It seeks to achieve this by identifying and articulating the skill and values of nurses' work with older people in all settings which provide continuous care.

Pauline Ford
Hazel Heath

National Frameworks and Values

Health and Social Policy Influences

Stuart Darby

Introduction

This chapter considers the way in which current legislation impacts upon the provision of residential and nursing home care in England and Wales. It will examine past social policy and recent developments that set out to shape and govern residential and nursing home services. Key issues regarding the provision of continuing care services are also raised.

There has been an increasing demand for care home provision in the last decade. The reasons include the increasing number of people over retirement age, changes in legislation and a reduction in local authority residential homes and National Health Service (NHS) continuing care beds (Hancock, 1995a). It is estimated that there are more than 10 million people above pension age in Britain, of whom 500 000 are in residential care. This represents a five-fold increase since the beginning of the century. By the year 2029, projected numbers of disabled older people will increase from the present 2 million to 6.5 million (Papworth, 1995).

The Registered Homes Act 1984, and later amendments, is the current major legislation that focuses upon the provision of residential and nursing home care (DHSS, 1984). More recently, the NHS and Community Care Act 1990 (DoH, 1990) has influenced the way in which older people access care homes and the way in which funding is provided. The government publication 'NHS responsibilities for Meeting Continuing Health Care Needs' (NHSE, 1995) confirms and clarifies NHS responsibilities for long-term care in England and Wales. It is anticipated that similar guidance will be issued for Scotland but in Northern Ireland it would seem that health authorities and social services have a well-established relationship. Readers are directed to the specific Government Acts for Scotland and Northern Ireland.

The growth of residential and nursing home care

In 1980, a discretionary power allowed, in theory, unlimited amounts of supplementary benefit to be paid to older people to enable them to be admitted to or remain in residential and nursing homes. It is suggested that this opened the door to independent home care providers. Attempts to control expenditure were made by imposing local limits on the amount of supplementary benefit payable. The number of residents in independent homes in England and Wales did, however, dramatically increase during this period (Parker, 1988). The greatest growth was in the private sector, which trebled between 1974 and 1984, whilst the voluntary sector increased only slightly. It is argued that this growth in residential and nursing home care also resulted from the fall in the number of NHS continuing care beds and the closure of long-stay institutions and mental illness hospitals. There was a positive side to the independent sector either stumbling across or exploiting central Government funds. Older people with limited income were able to place themselves in a home that was previously inaccessible. In some instances, public sector health and social service providers saw the advance of the independent sector as an opportunity to release resources that were otherwise tied up in their own residential care provision.

Until recently social policy has focused upon residential care provided by local authorities and NHS continuing care units, attempting to define their objectives in relation to hospitals on the one hand and community care on the other. In recent years however, the number of places in both public sector local authority homes and NHS continuing care units have been levelling off despite the rise in the number of people aged more than 75 years (Parker, 1988). The issues have also shifted from simply looking at the number of care home beds to quality issues and achieving improved consumer satisfaction (SSI, 1989 and 1993).

It is argued that the main reason for the White Paper Caring for People (DoH, 1989a) and the subsequent NHS and Community Care 1990 (DoH, 1990), was the need to do something about residential care and to look at alternative strategies to institutional care provision (Hudson, 1990).

An independent report (Wagner, 1988), was commissioned by the Government, to study the provision of residential care provided by the statutory, independent and voluntary sectors. It attempted to confront the notions that people could not normally be expected to live reasonable lives in such places; that few people want to go into residential care; that traditional forms of residential care have been ineffective; and that residential care is usually more expensive than possibly superior community care provision. Some of the recommendations of the Wagner Report were included in the subsequent NHS and Community Care Act (DoH, 1990) prompting the call to look at more appropriate domiciliary and community care. It also called for the promotion of independent sector care homes.

The need and demand for residential and nursing home care

Demand for long-term care comes from at least three sources: older people, their relatives and informal carers, and professionals. Many older people have a stereotyped view of the type and nature of long-term care.

This has been compounded recently by media reports of poor practice and standards of care (UKCC, 1994). Surveys show that many older people and their relatives would prefer care to be provided by a number of options including domiciliary care and care by relatives in order to retain personal independence, privacy and to avoid mixing with other 'uncongenial' people that would be anathema to their usual lifestyle. Residential and nursing home care is, however, considered by many to be the best option for older people with mental health problems. The advantages cited include the provision of safety and supervision, comfort and physical care, not having to worry about finances and reduction in loneliness (Wade, 1994).

The Registered Homes Act 1984

The Registered Homes Act 1984 (for England and Wales), and subsequent ammendments (DHSS, 1984), consolidates and amends previous legislation that governs residential and nursing home care provision. Part I of the Act refers to the registration and running of 'residential care homes' whilst Part II considers nursing homes and mental nursing homes.

Residential Care Homes (Part I): Part I of the Act requires that a 'residential care home' is registered with the local authority social services department. Residential care is defined as providing board and personal care. The Act defines 'disability' in relation to individuals who are blind, deaf, mute or substantially and permanently handicapped by illness, injury or congenital deformity or any other disability prescribed by the Secretary of State. Residential care homes are not required to be additionally registered with the local health authority, under Part II of the Act, unless applying for dual registration as a residential care home and a nursing and mental nursing home. District and community nurses are responsible for assessing and providing nursing care to residents.

Nursing and Mental Nursing Homes (Part II): Under Part II of the Act, these homes must be registered with the local health authority.

The main difference between Part I and Part II of the Act is that the nursing or mental nursing home must, at all times, be in the charge of a person who is a registered medical practitioner or a registered nurse. A qualified nurse must possess the qualifications specified by the Secretary of State. The number of nurses possessing such qualifications or to be on duty in the home may also be so specified. Mental nursing homes must state whether or not they intend to provide services for patients who may be detained under the Mental Health Act 1983, since this imposes an additional set of rules and regulations. Nursing care may be necessary where a client's general health deteriorates to a level that needs constant nursing care and where one or more of the following interventions are required during a twenty-four hour period:

- administration of medicine by injection,
- dressing to an open or closed wound,
- feeding requiring nursing skills,
- essential nursing care of the type given to people who are immobile or bedfast,
- intensive rehabilitation measures following surgery or associated with chronic debilitating disease, and
- management of complex psychological or aggressive states requiring nursing supervision.

Where homes wish to provide both residential and nursing care they must apply for dual registration. To achieve this, application for, and registration by, both the health and local authorities is necessary. The Royal College of Nursing, along with several other organisations is considering how homes registered to deliver both residential and nursing care might better meet the continuous needs of clients without their needing to move as dependency increases. This work is based on the fact that the needs of older people change over time. Although admitted to residential care, the older person may require episodes of nursing care or total nursing care. The current system of separate registration prevents continuity of care where nursing and health needs may change.

Annual registration fees are required to be paid to the registering authority. The fee is set by the Secretary of State. Certificates are issued to the registered home and as a general rule these should include the number, categories of resident, age and gender of residents who may be received in the home. Where a person is registered to receive patients detained under the Mental Health Act 1983, this must be specified in the certificate of registration. The certificate must be displayed in a prominent place within the home so that it can be clearly seen.

Under the Act, the local registration authorities are obliged to keep a record of all registered homes. This must be available for inspection and copies can be made of any entry made in the records.

The registration authority may refuse to register, or cancel the registration of, an individual in respect of a residential care home.

Inspection of homes

The respective registration authorities have a responsibility under the 1984 Act to appoint registration and inspection officers. From April 1991, registering authorities may request access to police records in respect of applicants for registration. This is not however a mandatory requirement. Under the Act, any person authorised by the Secretary of State may enter and inspect the premises and records. The regulations may prescribe inspection at set times during the year, but may also include inspection without appointment.

In the case of nursing and mental nursing homes, an authorised inspector may interview independently any patient residing in the home for the purpose of investigating a complaint or where the person has reason to believe that the patient is not receiving proper care. Where the person is a medical practitioner, they may examine the patient independently and may require the production of any medical records relating to treatment in the home. Many health authorities authorise a pharmaceutical officer to inspect nursing home arrangements to ensure that adequate arrangements for the storage, handling, record keeping, administration and disposal of medicines are in place.

It is argued that the Registered Homes Act 1984 is concerned mainly with adequacy and not quality (Smith, 1992). Swaffield (1990) considers that adequacy is not an appropriate measure in the current climate of ensuring quality services that meet individual demands and where control is supposed to take place by market forces. When local authorities place contracts with independent sector care homes or means test older people, the notion of consumer choice is removed and does not always protect those older people who are most likely to be highly dependent and vulnerable. Conversely, choice in relation to the old system of NHS continuing care beds and local authority residential accommodation was also diminished.

Where regulation, inspection and registration remains the responsibility of commissioning agencies' purchasing care, inspectors regulating premises may find that a conflict of interest exists in trying to uphold quality standards against a contract based on financial constraint. Although in some circumstances it may be appropriate for registration and inspection officers to monitor standards, there may be contention if the home fails to meet the criteria of adequacy. An inspector who requests improvements may need to take action against one of their own suppliers. The potential for public censure of the authority could compromise the inspector's position and be detrimental to the care of residents and patients. Inspectors may also be susceptible to pressure from 'would be' contractors to ensure that favourable reports are submitted (Royal College of Nursing, 1994).

National sandards, protocols and quality of service

The Royal College of Nursing (1994) calls for a national audit of the regulation of registered care homes and nursing homes. It recommends the setting up of a national audit as services, inspection and standards differ from one area to the next. The aim would be to achieve agreed national standards and protocols.

In addition, checks on owners and persons in charge of registered and nursing care homes are currently conducted in an ad hoc manner, with no standardised approach. There are currently no nationally agreed standards for determining inspectorate staffing levels and there are disparities across the country on the number of inspectors required. This often leads to minimum visits of two per annum. Often both visits are announced, rather than including unannounced visits. It is considered that this prevents inspectors from getting a true picture of care.

The fees for registration, set by the Government, have remained constant for the last four years and it is argued that these fees are insufficient to carry out the registration and inspection duties. As a result there may be too few inspectors, inadequate vetting of owners and individuals in charge and inadequate inspection of the premises and care given. Sufficient resources through registration fees payable to registering authorities could ensure that an appropriate number and quality of inspection officers are made available.

Costs are incurred by the registering authority inspectors for their inspection time and the provision of written reports, and expert advice is often sought from other professionals, such as pharmacists, psychiatric nurses and other therapists. This also needs to be paid for, particularly in the light of changes and a move to the NHS internal market.

Training

Finally, there is no consistent approach and continuity across the country in the way in which inspectors are trained or the way in which inspections are carried out. Different values of the registering local and health authorities may be reflected in the inspections and refusal or cancellation of registration. Minimum standards become the norm, again looking at adequacy rather than quality. Training packages were set up with Government funds in 1990 including the use of distance learning materials. These, however, were not mandatory but optional thereby reinforcing disparities across the country (Polytechnic of North London, 1990).

Registration

Most local and health authorities produce guidelines to assist prospective registered home owners in their application. Many follow the guidelines produced by the National Association of Health Authorities and Trusts (NAHAT, 1984). Authorities are, however, required to satisfy themselves of the fitness of the applicants to be registered. Again, there appears to be no standardised approach to ascertaining fitness and thus protecting vulnerable people. Disparities between assessing fitness included:

- requesting references, personal and professional,
- undertaking a police check,
- interviewing the applicant,
- checking finances,
- requesting a detailed curriculum vitae,
- requesting a statement about health,
- requesting a business plan,
- instituting a company search,
- checking professional qualifications of registered medical practitioners or registered nurses, and
- checking statements about health.

Given that registering authorities are able to cancel registration if it is proposed that the registered owner or person-in-charge is unfit, a standardised approach to vetting needs to be in place. A person whose application for registration is refused or revoked in one area can simply apply in another local authority or health authority (Swaffield, 1990).

The NHS and Community Care Act 1990

The NHS and Community Care Act 1990 (DoH, 1990) provides legislation for the role, function and responsibilities of local authority social service departments (SSDs) and Health Services in the provision of care to people in their own homes and elsewhere in the community. The main principles, originally set out in the White Papers 'Working for Patients' (DoH, 1989b) and 'Caring for People' (DoH, 1989a) include:

- the establishment of a health care market,
- increased consumer choice, independence and a range of options,
- a switch in emphasis from institution-based care to community based care,
- a combined approach of public, independent and voluntary agencies uniting to provide a comprehensive service, and
- provision of services that are flexible, sensitive and concentrate on those individuals and carers with the greatest need.

The establishment of a health care market

New funding arrangements were agreed with district health authorities and those GPs who opted to become fund holders. They became purchasers and were given a budget with which to contract, buy and achieve best value for money services, from a range of different agencies. The health authority then seeks bids from local hospitals, independent care agencies and community trusts to meet their contract requirements, including the type, range and quality of services required to meet the health needs of their given population. Providers of services, who submit and negotiate a plan which best matches the purchasers' requirements, obtain the business. This has introduced the element of competition within the health care market.

Consumer choice

The Government also produced the Patient's Charter (DoH, 1991), which sets out details of what consumers may expect in the delivery of health services. The charter established the first nine national standards, including access to information, reduced waiting time and access to services. The 'named nurse' concept requires that a named qualified nurse, health visitor or midwife will assume responsibility for a particular person's care.

The health service reforms have also initiated a change in the practice of GPs. The first of these gives GP's a major role in purchasing health care. A fund-holding practice controls its own budget, and buys health care that it cannot provide in-house on behalf of its patients. It is expected that those GPs who have elected to be non-fund holders will purchase through a system set up within the Family Health Service Authorities.

The second major change for GPs has been the issuing of contracts which are aimed at improving patient choice and standards of primary care. Since 1990, the contract demands that GPs meet targets for the early detection of unrecognised disease (screening) and offer regular health checks to specific groups of people, such as those aged over 75 years.

A switch in emphasis from institution-based care to community-based care

Community care: The main aim of the reforms was to enable people to remain in their own homes by promoting domiciliary, day and respite services.

Carers: To enable people to be able to continue to live in their own homes, services should be tailored to meet individual needs, including those of carers providing care for a dependent person at home.

Care management: In order for appropriate and comprehensive assessment to take place, a system of care management with an identified lead person within the local authority should be in place. The care manager has a responsibility for co-ordinating assessment, identification of needs, implementation of an agreed care plan and for evaluating and monitoring that care needs have been met.

Collaborative working: Although local authority social service departments are charged with the responsibility of ensuring that care management takes place, the legislation also recognises that a range of other caring agencies are required to ensure a comprehensive assessment of individual needs. Clarifying the role of other agencies in order to prevent confusion and encourage accountability is also a key component of the reforms.

Competition: In order to ensure that the widest choice of services, including residential and nursing home care, are made available, the legislation supports the view that independent, voluntary and non-profit-making organisations should be promoted and developed in addition to the existing public sector health and social services.

Channelling funds: A major part of the reforms introduced a new structure for funding social care with the aim of securing better value for money and promoting greater quality of care services. The provision of state funding for residential and nursing home care has been one of the most significant changes to impact upon older people under the legislation.

Key agency responsibilities

To achieve a combined and comprehensive approach of public, independent and voluntary agencies uniting services, the responsibilities of key agencies are set out as:

Local authority social service departments

● To make information accessible on the types of services available, the criteria for providing services, the assessment and complaints

procedures and the standards by which those procedures will be measured.
- To assess community care needs, negotiate and agree with other care agencies.
- To arrange and cost care packages and undertake regular review and evaluation of what clients and carers want, rather than providing traditionally services that are already in place.

Health authorities and NHS trusts

- To identify health care professionals to contribute to local authority led care assessments.
- To establish systems for feeding back information relating to health care needs.
- To ensure that appropriate health care is provided in relation to individual assessments.

General Practitioners

- To advise clients on the availability of local health and social services.
- To refer patients for community care assessments through the locally agreed procedure.
- To contribute to assessments and provide (with consent) professional advice and information where appropriate, on health issues that would affect a person's ability to remain in their own home.
- The implementation of GP practice funds and indicative prescribing budgets where GP's seek not to exceed indicative prescribing budgets laid down by FHSA (except with the consent of the authority or for good reasons.

Most commentators at the time agreed with the principles of the Act (Henwood, 1992). A jointly commissioned report (Bosanquet and Gray, 1989), argued that the last decade has missed the opportunity to develop an effective pattern of services and support for older people. The main impetus has been towards a further increase in long-term residential and nursing home care rather than a more community-based approach. Wadeson (1995) argues that the NHS and Community Care Act was a Government vehicle for steadily increasing privatisation of the NHS. Local authorities have been prevented from providing more than 15 per cent of direct care, thus further promoting the use of independent and independent sector care agencies. In 1981 the NHS lost 124 000 beds, transferring care to independent facilities and at the same time shifting the financial burden and responsibility on individuals and carers. Relatives and carers with chronically sick members of the family are reported to be the poorest in society (Rickford, 1993).

Vellenoweth (1990) argues that the stated aims of promoting independence were to be welcomed, but the changes were driven, in part, by the unplanned growth in social security support for people in independent residential and nursing home care, from £10 million in 1979 to £1000 million in 1989. A NAHA conference sought the views of a number of statutory, independent and voluntary agencies (NAHA, 1990). Some commentators thought that the rapid publication and initial timescale for implementation of the Act suggested that there was little time for discussion. Many felt that there was a need to set up a dialogue and have a real partnership with Government on resources, planning and training if people were to receive significantly better services.

The legislation was further considered to be descriptive rather than prescriptive as there was no national criteria or model upon which to base local systems for implementation (Laing, 1990). The Government countered this by stating that consultation would continue in parallel with implementation and that more formal guidance would be forthcoming. New Government guidelines go some way to addressing further consultation and guidelines (NHSE, 1995).

Concern was also expressed at the transfer of so much decision making to social service departments. As purchasing and quality-monitoring was to be placed with the local authority it was thought that there was a risk of falling standards. Care would be purchased on the basis of cost rather than quality where limited funding and resources were available. However, some agencies welcomed the fact that responsibility for the co-ordination of services would be placed with local authorities as this emphasised that the needs of older people, were not primarily medical. Some thought that health authorities were also at risk of losing out if they did not enter into a spirit of collaboration to ensure that their requirements were part of core specifications and that contracts were negotiated from the outset. In addition there was concern that care assessment and management is invested in social service departments with other agencies having a secondary and contributory role. Success would depend upon clear lines of responsibility being established and resources being used properly (Lewis, Dunn, and Vetter, 1994).

In response to the issues of creating competition between services, one agency felt that endless debate about the merits of public and independent provision were sterile and a waste of management time and energy. They considered that managers should be specifying their service requirements and judging providers on their ability to meet those requirements irrespective of whether they are in the public, independent or voluntary sectors.

In addition, NAHA stated that no voluntary agency would compete to run services on the cheap (NAHA, 1990). It considered that it was not realistic to expect the voluntary sector to take on a massive increase in services. Pluralism in care did not mean wholesale voluntarisation of mainstream services. At the same time there was also a need to safeguard the crucial role of the voluntary sector in advocacy and self-help. There was a danger that the advocacy role of the voluntary sector would be lost if organisations were paid and had to follow the requirements of the purchasing authority rather than act independently.

Many professionals and organisations were extremely sceptical about the potential effects of the Act. They thought that care in the community was probably underfunded as there was no ring fencing of specific money and it failed to guarantee even current levels of spending. There were also concerns that the increase in GP fund-holding may lead to some members of the community receiving a reduced service where rationing of health care may take place because of age or chronic illness (Heginbotham, 1992). It is also claimed that those GPs who are fund holders can jump the queue when negotiating care and that patients currently registered with GP fund-holding practices currently get a faster and better service (Martin, 1994).

Most agencies were concerned that there were to be no specific grants (except for the mentally ill) and that the Act stops short of guaranteeing additional resources for additional work to be carried out. These grants may also be diverted to other uses.

Vellenoweth (1990) considers that although the Act is strong on consumer choice, it fails to address the central question of ensuring that individuals and their carers have a major say in the assessment of need and the packaging of services. Assumptions were being made about individuals' preferences to remain in their own homes, and this could only be achieved if services are comprehensive and timely. Individuals may also still wish to opt for residential care. The Government believes that this should still be a positive choice, but that a place should only be secured if the assessment establishes a need for it as the whole or main component of care.

There were also concerns that a bureaucratic approach would introduce the birth of a remote specialist for assessment purposes. This may mean that block judgements are made without the intimate knowledge of the client or the neighbourhood. The speed at which the Act is being implemented may mean that professionals and older people may feel unduly pressured. This could lead to lack of choice for frail elderly and mentally infirm people, who, by definition, are the very people the Act is intended to help.

The legislation states that local authorities must set up arms length inspection units for their own and independent sector care homes. This is seen as clear response to the past inadequacies of local authorities' registration and inspection arrangements. Similar opportunities are not, however, being given to health authorities. This may be an implied credit, but raises the question of whether there is adequate recognition of the nursing home as a specialist resource within community care and without which 'Caring for People' is deficient.

Financing residential and nursing home care

Assessment of ability to pay

The local authority (SSD) is responsible for meeting the full cost of the care home. They will, however, assess the older person to see how much they can pay towards the costs by means testing or making a financial assessment according to national legislative criteria. Local authority means tests are similar to those carried out by the Department of Social Security for people claiming income support (DSS, 1993). Nursing homes now cost an average of between £300 and £500 a week, while the cost of home care ranges from £7.50 per hour on weekdays to almost £20 per hour on public holidays (Papworth, 1995).

Independent and independent sector homes: Most SSDs have a list of independent and voluntary homes that it has approved. If an older person wishes to go into a more expensive home, the difference in cost must be met by the older person or other family member. However, if there are no vacancies within a local authority's 'usual' care homes, the SSD must fund the difference. If an older person wishes to be a resident in a home that is outside the local authority, the rules on funding apply in the same way.

Means testing or financial assessments: To identify how much financial help an older person should receive, the local authority calculates all their weekly income (checking in the first instance that the older person is claiming all the benefits to which they are entitled) and subtracts it from the weekly fees of the home. If the care home fees exceed the older person's income, the difference in the balance is then paid at the discretion of the local authority.

The 1990 NHS and Community Care Act moved responsibility for assessing the care needs of older people to local authorities. Under the Act, those with assets and investments worth more than £8000, with the value of their houses taken into account, have to pay their own bills. For those with between £3000 and £8000 the state contribution is cut by £1 for every £250 of savings. Savings below £3000 are discounted. These sums were increased in the November 1995 Budget to £10 000 and £16 000, to be effective from April 1996. Also discounted are some types of income, such as the Disability Living Allowance, Mobility Component and any money from a relative or charity to pay for extras such as hairdressing or outings that are not included in the care home fees. During the first eight weeks of stay in residential care, the local authority does not have to carry out this charging assessment, but can use its discretion to charge whatever is reasonable. In 1992 an estimated 40 000 homes were sold to pay for care bills (Papworth, 1995).

Property ownership and its value can also be counted as part of savings, except where the stay in a care is home is expected to be temporary and less than 52 weeks. Although the older person cannot be forced to sell their home to pay for residential or nursing home care, the local authority can put a 'charge' upon it. This means that when the property is eventually sold they have first claim to any proceeds to pay off the money that the older person owes.

The value of the older person's home is not, however, counted as part of savings or capital where there is a spouse or partner residing there or another relative who is aged over 60 years or has a disability. Local authorities also have the discretion to discount the value of home ownership where there is a person aged 60 years or over living there or a younger person who has given up their own home to provide live-in care.

Payment of fees

The SSD may pay the care home directly and then collect the contribution from an older person or, if the older person agrees, the assessed amount may be paid directly by the older person and the balance topped up by the SSD.

Liable relatives: In some circumstances an older person's marital partner can be asked to contribute towards the cost of care. They are classed as a 'liable relative'. Usually, payment is voluntary and SSDs try to agree a fair amount. They can however apply for a court order if they think that the husband or wife can afford to pay something but is refusing to do so. No other family members, children, brothers and sisters or grandchildren can be made to contribute to care home costs.

Deprivation of assets: Some people may wish to give money away to relatives and friends, thus reducing their total savings or investments. This is known as deprivation of assets. If this occurs within six months of an older person being admitted to a home, and the local authority considers that this action has been a deliberate attempt to avoid paying for care, they can claim the money back from those who benefited. Even if the financial transfers took place more than six months ago, the older person can still be assessed as if they had the capital.

State benefits – Income Support: Income Support is a state benefit paid to those people whose income falls below a level set up by the Government. Residential Allowance can be claimed as an extra premium, by those older people entering independent or voluntary care homes where their income and savings are below the Government set level. It is intended to help with the cost of care in residential or nursing homes.

Those older people who reside in local authority homes can only claim income support if their personal income and savings is less than the State Retirement Pension. They cannot claim Residential Allowance.

State benefits – Disability Living Allowance, Care Component: The Care Component of the Disability Living Allowance stops after 28 days for people in local authority owned accommodation. It will also stop after 28 days for people in independent or voluntary residential care unless they are being funded wholly by themselves and/or a third party and they are not receiving Income Support or Housing Benefit or any funding from the local authority. The Care Component may stop sooner if, within the past 28 days, the claimant has already been in hospital or other 'special accommodation'. If the Disability Living Allowance ceases, then so will any premiums, such as Invalidity Benefit paid as a result of the Disability Living Allowance award. It should not, however, be withdrawn for older people with a terminal illness, residing in voluntary sector hospices. These rules also apply to those people receiving Attendance Allowance.

State benefits – Housing Benefit: No individual entering a residential care home for the first time after April 1993 will be eligible for housing benefit for that home. The only exception to this is where the residential accommodation is unregistered, such as certain types of hostel where lodging only (and not board) is provided.

Older people entering residential care temporarily who intend to return to their own home within 52 weeks can get Housing Benefit on their normal home as long as they fulfil the general rules for entitlement. This entitlement will stop if the normal home is rented out to someone else or it becomes evident that the older person does not intend to return home. People who are solely or mainly resident in residential care do not pay Council Tax.

Personal Expenses Allowance: Older people residing in residential and nursing homes are allowed a small Personal Expenses Allowance (£13.10 in April 1994) which can be used by them to purchase, for example, clothes, toiletries and other individual personal items.

Preserved rights: Although older people who were residents before April 1993 have preserved rights, if they move out of a home for 13 weeks or more or spend 52 weeks in hospital, protection ceases. If residential care is needed again, the new arrangements outlined above are applied.

NHS responsibilities for meeting continuing health care needs

In 1995, the National Health Service Executive produced guidance on NHS, local authorities and GP fund holders responsibilities for meeting continuing care needs (NHSE, 1995). The guidance tends to be descriptive rather than prescriptive. It states that all agencies must collaborate, consult and agree locally on their respective responsibilities for providing a full range of services to meet the needs of their continuing care population. Individuals cited in this category include those people being discharged from hospital and those who require continuing in-patient care, rehabilitation, palliative health care, respite health care, community health services support, specialist transport and specialist or intensive health care support.

The guidance states that health authorities must have final policy and eligibility criteria in place by April 1996. Eligibility criteria must be set out to identify those people accessing continuing care provided by local authorities and those provided by health authorities.

Under existing guidelines NHS patients cannot be placed in an independent, nursing or residential home against their will if it means that they or their relatives will be responsible for paying the fees. The Government's latest guidance, however, gives health authorities and hospitals the right to 'take account of the needs of other patients in determining how long the person can continue to occupy an NHS bed'. They do, however, have the right to refuse to be discharged from NHS care into a nursing or residential home. Other options should be explored but, if these options have been rejected, it may be necessary for the hospital, in consultation with the local health authority and local authority SSD, to implement discharge to the patient's own home or alternative accommodation with a package of health and social care within the options and resources available. A charge may be payable by the person for the social care element of the package (Brindle, 1995).

Whilst the debate about health care and social care has been in existence for some time and the guidance is well overdue (Hancock, 1995b), they raise a number of issues in relation to the future of all forms of continuing care.

Eligibility criteria: The guidance proposes that individual health authorities together with local authorities should decide who is eligible for NHS-funded long-term care by defining and agreeing eligibility criteria. As there will be no national criteria, those who need continuing care will not know what to expect. In addition, their choice as consumers (underpinning the NHS and Community Care Act) will be reduced in the type, range and provision of care that they may access.

National equity of services: There are also fundamental concerns about the fair and equitable provision of continuing care. There may be major geographical variations in eligibility criteria. Older people may therefore not receive free NHS care, or be subject to means-tested care, dependent upon which hospital they attend or where they live.

Funding: The dangers here are twofold. Older people may be refused care by local authorities who have run out of community care funds (Cassidy, 1995) and/or refused care by a health authority as they do not meet the eligibility criteria. The eligibility criteria may be set according to the funding and resources allocated to health and local authorities, rather than being based upon need and demand.

In setting out a distinction between medical needs (health authority responsibility) and social needs (local authority responsibility), health authority care will be free at point of use. However, if a local authority places its contracts for long-term care with independent residential or nursing homes, older people will be subject to means testing. This guidance makes it more likely therefore that older people will be expected to pay for previously free nursing home care.

Finally, the guidance takes no account of, and fails to acknowledge, the complex and essential activity of nurses and other health therapists (Hancock, 1995a). These services can be costly and are essential to health and well being for older people who have chronic or debilitating illnesses. Decisions about which authority is responsible will therefore be crucial on the basis that there is a distinction between health and social care.

Conclusion

Demographic changes: Great Britain has the highest proportion of over 65s in the European Community. By the year 2001, the number of people over 75 years of age is likely to grow by 42 per cent whilst the 85+ age group will more than double. Older people make seven to eight times the demands on health and welfare services than the rest of the population. Between 1979 and 1986 residential care escalated by 190 per cent with about 45 per cent of those in independent or voluntary homes funded through social security funds care (Leathard, 1991). This places pressure on financing and resourcing health and social care. In 1981, 96.6 per cent of people of pensionable age lived in independent households. Local authorities have increasingly been unable to meet the rising demands for residential and nursing homes. They have since been mandated to promote the use of independent sector care for older people (DoH, 1990).

Legislative changes: The NHS and Community Care Act (1990) aimed to introduce a set of principles that would help in achieving and ensuring unity between different care providers and those people who were purchasing care on the behalf of older people. Challis et al. (1988) show that joint approaches are problematical and difficult to achieve, although essential for managing the increasing complexity of care provision. This pressure is inextricably linked with joint financing, separate management systems, training and policies between local authorities, health services and social security funding. The latest National Health Service Executive guidance on NHS responsibilities (NHSE, 1995) compounds these issues by attempting to define health and social care. The main concerns are that the needs of older people often change. Setting local demarcation lines of responsibility may leave them more vulnerable and unable to access or choose the type of care that they would like or need. The legislation within the Registered Homes Act 1984 is overdue for review and evaluation. Any future review or change needs to address quality of services and quality of life, rather than simply looking at the number of beds.

The future of residential, nursing and NHS continuing care

The current thrust to ensure that continuity of care for older people in residential and nursing homes is achieved through 'single ticket' (or dual registration) homes has many implications. For older people it will provide the safety net of ensuring that continuity of care is provided. Nursing care will be available on a twenty-four hour basis for those people who require it, rather than visits from district nurses to those people currently in single registration residential homes.

As a result, the role, function, skill and status of nurses working with older people in continuing care must be recognised and valued (Royal College of Nursing, 1993), despite that fact that latest 1995 Government guidelines fail to take this into account (NHSE, 1995). In the United States of America a shift to nursing home care led to increased dependency in nursing homes. As a result, teaching nursing homes linked to universities, were established. These have shown great success in serving as education centres for all health care staff, permitting worthwhile research to be undertaken and upgrading clinical care and standards in a co-ordinated and worthwhile fashion (Grady and Earll, 1990). This model exists where a climate of private and independent sector care also prevails.

There needs to be continuing discussion and debate about the provision of independent sector versus NHS continuing care, and the fact that means-tested care may affect access and choice for older people. This, however, is no less important than issues about the quality of care provision and the rights and value that we place upon older people in society.

REFERENCES

Brindle, D. (1995) Hospitals can send the elderly home. *The Guardian*. 24 February.

Cassidy, C. (1995) RCN warns of long-term care 'lottery' for older people. *Nursing Standard*, **91**(20) 17 May, p. 7.

Challis L. and Baitlett H. (1987) Old and Ill, private nursing homes for elderly people, Research Paper 1, Age concern Institute of Gerontology.

Department of Health (1989a) Caring for People: Community Care in the Next Decade and Beyond, Cmnd 849, London: HMSO.

Department of Health (1989b) Working for Patients. London: HMSO.

Department of Health (1990) The NHS and Community Care Act. London: HMSO.

Department of Health (1991) The Patient's Charter. London: HMSO.

Department of Health and Social Security (1984) The Registered Homes Act 1984. England and Wales. London: HMSO.

Department of Social Security (1993) Care in the community: Changes in income support and other social security benefits from 1st April 1993. Leaflet SSCC1. London: HMSO.

Grady, M.J. and Earll, J.M. (1990) Teaching physical diagnosis in the nursing home. *American Journal of Medicine*, **88**(5), 519–521.

Hancock, C. (1995a) What is Long Term Care? *Health Service Journal*, 5 January, p. 15.

Hancock, C. (1995b) What Price Long Term Care? *Nursing Standard*, 17 May, **9**(34), p. 46.

Heginbotham, C. (1992) Leading for health: Responses: Rationing. *British Medical Journal*, **304**, 22 February, pp. 496–499.

Henwood, M. (1992) Through A Glass Darkly: Community Care and Elderly People. Research Report No. 14. London: King's Fund Institute.

Hudson, B. (1990) Yes, but will it work? (Collaboration between local and health authorities crucial for community care). *Health Services Journal*, **100**(1) 169–70.

Laing, W. (1990) Grey Cloud Hides A Silver Lining. *Community Care*, 26 July.

Leathard, A. (1991) *Health Care Provision: Past, Present and Future*, pp. 112–114. London: Chapman and Hall.

Lewis, P.A, Dunn, R.B. and Vetter, N.J. (1994) NHS and Community Care Act 1990 and discharges from hospital to private residential and nursing homes. *British Medical Journal*, **309**, 2 July, pp. 28–29.

Martin, A. (1994) Community Care: the end of first term report. *Care of the Elderly*, April, p. 138.

NAHA (1990) *National Association of Health Authorities News*, January, Issue No. 134.

NAHAT (1984) National Association of Health Authorities: Registration and Inspection of Nursing Homes.

NHSE (1995) NHS Responsibilities for Meeting Continuing Health Care Needs. HSG(94) NHS Executive.

Papworth, J. (1995) Elderly Infirm losing state safety net. *The Guardian*. 20 May.

Parker, R.A. (1988) Residential Care for Elderly People. In I. Sinclair (ed.) *Residential Care: The Research Reviewed*. National Institute for Social Work.

Polytechnic of North London (1990) Making Sense of Inspection: Registered Homes Act 1984: Training Course for Registration and Inspection Staff. Polytechnic of North London.

Rickford, F. (1993) Long-stay Beds for Elderly Cut by 40%. *The Guardian*, 5 August.

Royal College of Nursing (1993) Older People and Continuing Care – The Skill and Value of The Nurse. Royal College of Nursing.

Royal College of Nursing (1994) An Inspector Calls: The Regulation of Private Nursing Homes and Hospitals. Royal College of Nursing.

Smith, J. (1992) Home rules: Choosing between residential and community care for elderly clients. *Social Work Today*, **23**, 16 January, p. 23.

SSI (1989) Homes are for Living in. Department of Health/Social Services Inspectorate. HMSO.

SSI (1993) Inspection of Local Authority Care for Mentally Disorded People. Department of Health/Social Services Inspectorate. London: HMSO.

Swaffield, L. (1990) Monitoring Muddles. *Nursing Times*, **86**(45), 7 November, pp. 31–32.

Townsend, P. (1962) *The Last Refuge*. Routledge and Kegan Paul.

UKCC (1994) Professional Conduct – occasional report on standards of nursing in nursing homes. London: United Kingdom Central Council for Nursing, Midwifery and Health Visiting.

Vellenoweth, C. (1990) Caring for people. *National Association of Health Authorities News*, January, Issue No. 134. p. 8.

Wade, B (1994) The changing face of community care. Daphne Heald Research Unit, Royal College of Nursing.

Wade, B. Sawyer, L. and Bell, J. (1983) Dependency with Dignity: Different Care Provision for the Elderly. Occasional Papers on Social Administration No. 68, Bedford Square Press and the National Council for Voluntary Organisations, London.

Wadeson, B. (1995) War on the weak. *Nursing Standard*, **9**(18), 25 January, p. 54.

Wagner Report (1988) Residential Care: A Positive Choice. Volumes I and II. London: HMSO.

2

Meeting the Needs of the Locality

Helen Peace

Introduction

Locality planning involves the assessment of need. It aims to develop locally sensitive health and social care provision in order to ensure the efficiency, effectiveness and equality of services for people who live in the local community.

Several key policy changes in recent years have resulted in the development of locality planning. The context in which locality planning takes place, how it is carried out and influencing factors will be discussed in this chapter, which also seeks to explore some of the presenting opportunities for care homes.

Community care

The Community Care Act (1990) covers England and Wales, amends the previous NHS Scotland Act (1978) but does not fully apply to Northern Ireland. The parts which do apply have been incorporated into the Health and Personal Social Services (NI) Order 1991.

The community care reforms gave local authorities the lead for community care. The new arrangements seek to promote a collaborative approach of co-operation between agencies so that a comprehensive service can be offered for both users and carers.

Users' and carers' centrality in service provision requires a radical change in culture. The first challenge is to listen and to hear what the users of the service are asking for. The Community Care Act aims to provide a shift in influence favouring users and their carers (DoH, 1992). It creates a planning framework in which agencies must start to work much more closely together, and places greater emphasis on consultation and collaboration at every level. It seeks to address inconsistencies between community care policies and social security arrangements for funding residential and nursing home care by transferring the care element of this funding to local authorities.

All authorities involved in community care should be involved in the introduction of a specific community care charter (DoH, 1994). Charters should be developed locally to reflect the locally planned and delivered community care service. Local charters should be developed with and for local people, particularly those who use, or may need to use, community care services, and the people who care for them.

The United Kingdom is now a multi-ethnic, multi-cultural society and the National Health Service and local community charters should reflect this. Many services provided have been insensitive and inappropriate, and access impeded by cultural and language barriers between health professionals and their black and ethnic majority clients (Jayaratnam, 1993).

The Patients' Charter (DoH, 1991) has emphasised the need for a National Health Service which is responsive to patients' needs. It is an integral part of the important shift towards consumer empowerment which affects primary and secondary care. The Charter emphasies the need for respect for privacy, dignity and religious and cultural beliefs. It is necessary to identify what these aspects of the Charter mean. Service provision should aim to meet the health and social care needs of the diverse group of older people in each locality.

Locality planning

Working for Patients (DoH, 1989) and the NHS and Community Care Act itself, (DoH, 1990), present opportunities for purchasers to improve health care delivery. The concept of an internal market has been introduced with purchasers contracting with providers for the services which they wish to purchase. One aim is to ensure that health service units compete against one another for funds, thus providing a powerful motivator to improve the efficiency and effectiveness of the service.

The purchasers/commissioners should assess the health needs of the local population and purchase health care services accordingly. Purchasers/commissioners will negotiate with competing provider units to sign contracts for services at agreed prices.

The main purchasers in the internal market are health authorities and GP fund holders. The main providers will include acute hospital services and community services.

Social services have the lead responsibility for ensuring the provision of appropriate community social care. The prime task is to identify the needs and achieve care in the community at, or close to, people's homes by securing and operating integrated care through effective collaboration between local authorities and other organisations inside and outside the NHS.

The DSS works with housing departments and associations to promote appropriate living environments for older people by housing adaptation and renovation, and by the identification of the need for residential and nursing homes for the very frail and dependent older person.

The role of commissioning and purchasing

Commissioning teams are responsible for assessing the needs of the local population and therefore assess what services need to be available. Purchasing teams then make a selection as to what the priorities are for the locality in terms of assessed health need, available or potential provision, and what funds are available. They then contract with various purchasers to secure provision of the service at the most cost-effective price.

Locality purchasing aims to develop locally sensitive health purchasing in order to ensure effectiveness, efficiency and equity for the residents of the locality. The commissioning team should have an understanding of the locality and its influences on health and illness. They are responsible for ascertaining the numbers in particular age groups within the locality. This is called a local population study and should identify the numbers of older people living within the locality, and where they live. It should also highlight any particular characteristics which influence health, for example, numbers living alone or former work patterns which have had an influence on health status.

Information on current service provision is collected by evaluating service accessibility, availability and responsiveness. The acceptability of the services to all potential and actual users, for example GP practices, day hospitals, day care and drop-in centres is also ascertained. The commissioning team looks at which services need to be developed in order to meet the needs of the people living in each area of the locality. Public transport routes and timetables, main roads and other barriers which affect siting of services need to be taken into account and wheelchair access to services needs to considered.

The commissioning team also seeks to identify any particular ethnic groups who are likely to have specific needs. Other groups may have known special needs because of their housing situation or general poverty. Having identified that there is, for example, a community of ageing Afro-Caribbeans, the commissioning team should ascertain what their specific needs are and how to plan for them.

If we accept that socio-economic factors are key determinants of health status then good practice suggests that planning is a collaborative event between health and social commissioning teams, and also local members of the community acting as their representatives, for example, voluntary organisations and Community Health Councils.

Community Health Councils were set up as local independent bodies in 1974 to represent the interests, in the health service, of the public in each district. The primary purpose of the CHC is to influence the nature of health care provision and to monitor its quality on behalf of the local population. They also identify services which are needed but not yet provided. Community Health Councils are statutory bodies and have rights to information, to be consulted, and to meet with health authorities, trusts and local authorities. They participate in debate and discussion on national and regional policies which have an impact on the local community, and they inform the public, relevant statutory bodies and voluntary organisations on key health issues and choices. They are being asked to participate in the decisions that NHS purchasers need to make because of the gap between the resources available and the need for health care.

The goal is to improve the health and social well-being of the local community. A competitive internal market has been established with many hospitals and community units seeking to adapt business planning and marketing methods from the world of commerce (Teasdale, 1992).

Purchasers act as agents for the public by assessing people's health needs and developing local strategies for improving health. It is their responsibility to purchase services, targeting resources through the contracts they have with providers of health care.

Purchasers should give early long-term direction to the providers in order for them to have sufficient time to plan desired changes to the way in which services are delivered. In any locality there will be differing needs because of the age range, and funding will need to be targeted appropriately, taking into account the estimated rise of the numbers of older people living in the community.

The role of the providers

Providers in the NHS work closely with purchasers to secure services which meet the needs identified by purchaser contracts. They are expected to be responsive to the needs of their patients in delivering high-quality and cost-effective care. Providers are also responsible for ensuring effective co-operation across service, education and research.

The providers are the units which actually give treatment and care to patients. They may be hospital or community units, and may offer any type of service which aims to meet health and social care needs. Both health and social service providers exist in any one locality. They will provide a mix of services which is likely to include, for example, hospitals, day hospitals, day centres and domiciliary care. Statutory, private and voluntary sectors are all likely to be providers. Community care provision, for example, will include some or all of the following:

- home care,
- aids and equipment for daily living,
- day, residential and nursing home care,
- chiropody at home,
- laundry services, and
- meals on wheels.

These are commonly provided by the local authority, private and voluntary sectors.

The NHS, in the form of Trusts and GP fund holders are likely to offer all or some of the following:

- community nursing services,
- community cardiac support service,
- health promotion,

- equipment provided by the NHS,
- physiotherapy,
- speech and language therapy,
- occupational therapy,
- chiropody,
- continence advice, and
- support/counselling.

Some services are provided by social services and housing working together; for example, housing adaptations provided through housing authorities and allocation of accommodation for people with care needs. This would include sheltered and specially adapted housing.

Day care

One particular service which I believe has key potential are day hospitals. They can form a valuable service for older people. With minimal exceptions, every health district has one or two. A recent report (National Audit Office, 1994) concluded that day hospital care is an important component of community health services which assists older people to live independent lives in their own homes. A day hospital provides services including assessment, planning, implementation and evaluation of care for older people living in the community who require some form of medical, nursing or rehabilitative care on a daily basis. Health education is promoted to the people who are interested. This aspect of health care can take place on a one to one or group basis and can be accomplished wherever there is a group of older people. Psychogeriatric day hospitals provide services for older people with mental health needs which may include such conditions as depression or dementia.

A further report (Research Unit of the Royal College of Physicians and the British Geriatric Society, 1994) suggests that maintainence of independence, provision of respite services and social care and support need careful consideration reflecting local need and circumstances. The report supports the need for day hospitals for maintainence of functional ability in older people, particularly if the need cannot be met by other service providers. Such decisions clearly require joint planning between health and community care purchasers.

Before contracting with a day hospital or any provider, purchasers will question what is being provided and if this is the most appropriate arena for health and social care. Health and social joint funding could provide a model of day care for the older person, and an environment that could respond to all the needs of an individual person. Rigid boundaries should be broken down to enable the older person to have access to health and social care.

Opportunities for care homes

Such detail on day care has been offerred in the hope that you will consider the value of day care provision in a home. Opportunities exist for entrepreneurial nursing homes to provide a model of day care that offers the resource of nursing, support and advice to older people living in the community. It could be adopted by the community in which it is located and provide a service to the older residents of the area.

Meals could be provided to non-residents on a daily basis. This would give an opportunity for the nurse to discuss what the older person is eating and offer advice on a healthy eating pattern, particularly to someone living alone. Medication could be discussed and advice given as appropriate. Chiropody, laundry and hairdressing facilities could be of benefit to the local population and bathing using the specialised equipment would be of benefit to the local population. Medication could be discussed and advice given as appropriate.

It is recognised that bathing is an essential part of community care (RCN, BASW, 1993) and, particularly if equipment is required, the bathing could be offered in a care home where nursing expertise is available. A bath provides an opportunity for the older person to discuss concerns and it gives the nurse the occasion to assess the functional ability and condition of the skin of the older person.

Social interaction is valued by many older people, especially someone who has had a family and is now living alone. We should not underestimate the problems that boredom and the lack of mental and social stimulation can have on the health and well-being of the older person.

Day care in a home can benefit people living in the community, provide stimulation in many forms and also give relief to informal carers for a period during the week.

Respite care

One important initiative for carers is short term respite care. Traditionally such respite has been provided in a hospital setting on pre-agreed terms such as six weeks at home and two weeks in respite care. In some areas this form of assistance is neither easily available nor very flexible. Carers express concern about the need for respite which is consistant with the needs of the individual as well as the carers. Any service offered therefore should reflect as closely as possible the normality of the individual's life routines and activities. Such care can be provided in the individuals own home, in a care home, or, if absolutely necessary in a hospital setting. For those with dementia in particular, the traditional form of two weeks of respite care, sometimes in different venues can leave them feeling more confused and disorientated than they were before. If day and respite care is in the same location every time, and the home located close to the person's own home, familiar staff would lessen anxiety for both the older person and their carer.

Community nurses are attached to GPs' practices and provide professional nursing care and support in collaboration with GPs, social services, voluntary agencies and carers. District nurses undertake nursing assessment. They also plan, implement and review nursing care for people living in the community. Within the community nursing team there are people who specialise in particular services, for example, the Continence Advisory Service. The main aim of this service is to promote continence and assess, treat and manage incontinence. They work within the health care team to advise and support clients and carers, as well as educating and training other professional colleagues.

Community cardiac support services can offer continuing professional support and advice to those who have been discharged from coronary care units or medical wards. Community therapists provide a service aimed at promoting maximum independence in mobility, self-care and communication difficulties. They assess and advise on equipment and modifications to buildings and surrounding areas, for example, wheel-chairs and the requirement for suitable access.

Social services' primary task is to support people in a locality by identifying their needs, by representing their interests, by using resources to provide and obtain services and by working with other agencies and organisations for the benefit of people living in the community. It is also the task of social services to support people within their own homes through the provision of social care services. They are both providers and purchasers, and take the lead role in assessment for community care. When the needs are health-related nurses must be involved in the assessment process. Social services are providers of domiciliary and residential care but they will also purchase this, and nursing home care, from the private sector.

They will assess needs on an individual basis, for example, laundry services, and purchase from a local source. Social services will give operational grants to bodies of people to provide a service for the community, for example, meals on wheels.

Social service departments have no powers to provide ordinary domestic houses, so it is necessary for them to have links with local housing authorities, housing associations and private providers of homes for older people.

Future service provision will need to reflect the estimated rise of older people in the community (OPCS, 1991), and housing is clearly important. Providing repairs and adaptations are vital elements in helping older people to remain in homes of their own (Henwood, 1991). There is a need for close links between local and health authorities, housing and private and voluntary agencies if the needs of the local population are to be met.

Homes can be providers of care on a permanent, intermittent or day care basis. They play an important part in meeting people's health and social needs. Whatever the successes of community care, some people will always need more support than can reasonably be provided in their own homes or in sheltered housing. The informed choices of the older person should always predominate in discussions regarding moving from their own home into a care home.

Levels of owner occupation and hence of capital assets, and also of other wealth (such as personal and occupational pensions) will continue to increase among older people. The growth of privately financed care will be dependent on how far older people are willing to spend assets they might otherwise bequeath (Henwood, 1991), or on funding from social services following a detailed health and social assessment of the individual person.

Care homes have the opportunity to expand their facilities as providers by offering, to older people and the purchasers of health and social care, expertise for people living in their locality. As an example, they could provide facilities for out-patient and therapy clinics. It would appear to be more efficient and effective, in many instances, to take the expertise into the community than have large groups of older people travelling to a district general hospital, often by hospital transport, for a 20 minute consultation.

Homes can act as a resource to the locality, providing expert advice and information on health, social and domestic issues. A vast range of equipment is available to help make everyday living easier for the older person, such as, information on benefits, alarm schemes, equipment, talking books, safety in the home, transport schemes and caring for pets. Care homes are ideally placed to offer this kind of information and advice.

Daily attendance at a venue rehabilitation, nursing care and social interaction will help the individual person to live as active a life as possible in the community.

Reminiscence activities could be organised. This would not only provide an opportunity for older people to be listened to but also allows individuals to express feelings and emotions. This may be particularly useful for those older people who are isololated in their community living (McCourt, 1994). The care home offering advice on continence aids and a laundry service to the locality could help older people and their carers to cope with incontinence problems.

Many older people are now using private agencies for home care. A home could offer training of such care workers who are giving direct care, for example, moving, lifting and handling techniques.

The role of the GP fund holder

Fund holders are those GPs who have put themselves forward to hold public money to use directly to buy services for their patients. The agreed budget for a fund holder is deducted from the total sum of money allocated to the health authorities. The fund holders can negotiate over quality and price issues as they control some of the funds the providers need to run their service. The fund holders are independent contractors and can purchase a hospital consultant's time to provide an out-patient clinic in the GP practice or other suitable facility.

Individual assessment

The Community Care Act requires the local authorities to carry out care assessments should they consider a person in need of community services. In order to guarantee holistic evaluation of each older person, this assessment should be jointly managed by health and social services. Effective community care for frail older people depends critically upon the integration and co-ordination of health and social care. One immediate benefit should be an end to the random nature of the way in which older people, who can no longer cope alone, find themselves being admitted to nursing or residential homes. In the long term, it is hoped that many more increasingly dependent people will be able to remain in their own homes with support from health and social services.

There are nurses working in the community to support people who choose to live in their own homes. Since April 1995, people can expect to be consulted about a convenient time for a visit, within a two-hour time band (DoH, 1994). A visit from the community nursing team will occur within four hours if the referral is urgent, within two working days if the referral is non-urgent and by appointment on the day asked for if the community nurses have more than 48 hours' notice.

Carers and voluntary organisations

Informal carers are people who look after relatives or friends who, because of disability, illness or the effects of old age, cannot manage at home without help. Popular belief suggests that the vast majority of carers are women. However, in 1990 of the 6.8 million carers, 2.9 million were men and 3.9 million were women (OPCS, 1992). Carers themselves need advice and support because of the extra responsibilities they are undertaking. Community care is intended to help frail, disabled and ill people to stay in their own home. Yet many of these people are still not receiving the help and support they need and to which they are entitled. Many carers are unaware that they can ask for an assessment for the person they care for and have their needs considered. Some useful organisations and their activities are outlined below:

The Carers' National Association is a voluntary organisation with branches and local offices throughout the UK. They give information, support and advice to people who are caring at home.

The Citizens Advice Bureau can advise on problems relating to help and care at home and can offer guidance for further contact if they are unable to help. They provide the largest advice service in the country.

The British Red Cross provides a range of services throughout the United Kingdom, including loans of mobility aids, a transport and escort service and, in some parts of the UK, a home from hospital scheme and day care services.

Crossroads is a national organisation with approximately 250 local schemes affiliated to the national office. The money for the schemes comes from a core fund from a service agreement with social services, donations, fund raising activities and occasionally from the person requiring their services. The Crossroads care attendant aims to complement, not replace, the services provided by district nurses, home carers, meals on wheels, etc. They have a role to undertake work an informal carer would normally carry out, for example, personal hygiene, assistance in the management of continence of bladder and bowels, assistance with feeding, and light domestic duties. However any invasive procedure are not undertaken by the care attendants. This is currently being discussed at national level.

Age Concern England, Wales, Northern Ireland and Scotland consist of a network of over 1100 independent groups throughout the UK. These provide a range of vital local services which may include information and advice, day care, visiting services, lunch clubs, over 60s' clubs, and hospital discharge services. Centrally Age Concern publish information on many subjects relating to ageing, including health, death and bereavement, financial and legal matters.

The Chest, Heart and Stroke Association works for the prevention of chest, heart and stroke illnesses and provides sympathetic and practical help. The existence of a Stroke Club in the locality provides a meeting place for the mutual benefit of people who have had a stroke and their carers. For most people the club is an important social outlet, particularly as they can converse with people who have similar problems.

The Parkinson's Disease Society concentrates on the particular problems caused by the disease. Next to arthritis and strokes, Parkinson's disease probably poses more problems with mobility than any other disease of the locomotor system. Activity and encouragement within the older person's capabilities are important. Both at head office and in the local branches the society has a wealth of knowledge and experience to work with people in solving problems, offering support, friendship and advice.

Counsel and Care, a voice for older people, aims to make available advice and practical help to older people and their carers. It provides grants where possible and information on services and benefits, and advises those working with older people. It sets out to promote the positive image of older people. They comment and campaign on a variety of social policy issues, for example, age discrimination in welfare benefits.

Help the Aged works to improve the quality of life of older people, particularly those who are frail, isolated or poor. The charity has a range of free advice leaflets on welfare and disability benefits, money matters, home safety and health.

Pensioner Action Groups are pressure groups run by senior citizens to lobby Government on issues relating to equity in opportunity. Some members have expressed a fear of being discharged from hospital too early and the care in the community being 'rationed'. Many fear they will be living isolated lives and will not have the opportunity to live life to their full potential because of lack of knowledge on facilities available.

These represent the vast number of organisations that are available to assist and advice older people.

Conclusion

The current climate of community care with its emphasis on planning and provision within the locality potentially widens opportunities for care homes to extend the range of services they offer. This chapter has described how an established care home can diversify to provide a range of services for older people and offer the resource of nursing expertise and support.

There appears to be a gap in meeting the needs of the older person living in the community, particularly at night and during weekends. Nursing homes could fill this gap. The majority of carers cope during the day often with help from health or social services. But the need is often greater at night at at the weekends when these services are very limited.

The opportunities for care homes to be part of community services for the older person are immense. It will take planning and change, and a willingness to be responsive and flexible.

Nurses working in care homes have the opportunity to influence the quality of life, health care and social needs of older people, their families and carers. This can take place within a care home and as part of an outreach service. Such initatives present opportunities and challenges for nurses who wish to demonstrate their creative and responsive approaches to meeting the health care needs of older people.

Useful contacts

Carers' National Association, 20/25 Glasshouse Yard, London EC1A 4JS. Tel: 0171 490 8818.

National Association of Citizens Advice Bureaux, Myddelton House, 115-123 Pentonville Road, London N1 9LZ. Tel: 0171 833 2181.

The British Red Cross Society, 9 Grosvenor Crescent, London SW1X 7EJ. Tel: 0171 235 5454.

Association of Crossroads Care Attendant Schemes Ltd., 10 Regent Place, Rugby, Warwickshire CV21 2PN. Tel: 01788 573653.

Age Concern England, Astral House, 1268 London Road, London SW16 4ER. Tel: 0181 679 8000.

The Chest, Heart and Stroke Association, CHSA House, Whitecross Street, London EC1Y 8JJ. Tel: 0171 490 7999.

The Parkinson's Disease Society, 36 Portland Place, London. Tel: 0171 255 2432.

Counsel and Care, Twyman House, 16 Bonny Street, London NW1 9PG. Tel: 0171 485 1566.

Help the Aged, St James's Walk, London EC1R 0BE. Tel: 0171 253 0253.

References

Department of Health (1989) Working for Patients. London: HMSO.
Department of Health (1990) The NHS and Community Care Act. London: HMSO.
Department of Health (1991) The Patient's Charter. London: HMSO.
Department of Health (1992) Community Care: Managing the Cascade of Change. London: HMSO.
Department of Health (1992) The Community Revolution, Social Services and Community Care. London: HMSO.
Department of Health (1994) A Framework for Local Community Care Charters in England. London: HMSO.
Henwood, M. (1991) Through a Glass Darkly, Community Care and Elderly People. King's Fund Institute, Research Report No. 14. London.
Jayaratnam, R. (1993). The Need for Cultural Awareness. In A. Hopkins and V. Bahl, (ed.) *Access to Health Care for People from Black and Ethnic Minorities*, pp. 11–20, Royal College of Physicians.
McCourt, V. (1994) Cherish the Memory. *Nursing Times*, **90**, 63.
National Audit Office (1994) National Health Service Day Hospitals for Elderly People in England. London: HMSO.
Office of Population Censuses and Surveys (1993) Persons Aged 60 Years and Over, Great Britain, (1991 Census). London: HMSO.
Office of Population Censuses and Surveys (1992), General Household Survey: Carers in 1990 London: HMSO.
Research Unit of the Royal College of Physicians and the British Geriatric Society (1994). Report, Geriatric Day Hospitals. Royal College of Physicians, London.
Royal College of Nursing and British Association of Social Workers (1994). Bathing: an Essential Service, London: RCN.
Teasdale, K. (1992) *Managing the Changes in Health Care*. Wolfe Publishing Ltd.

3

Professional Nursing Issues

Abigail Masterson

Introduction

Nurses working with older people in care home settings aim to provide effective, appropriate, high quality care. This chapter deals with a selection of professional issues which are pertinent to the provision and delivery of such care. It is impossible to include everything, and the discussion must necessarily be brief as each issue could merit a whole chapter in itself. Some of the issues will be developed further in other chapters, and suggestions for additional reading and useful contacts are included at the end of the chapter.

The chapter opens with a definition of quality, discusses a variety of possible strategies for assuring quality, and outlines the factors involved. An explanation of the statutory body for nursing and its impact on nursing practice with regard to accountability, responsibility, supervision and delegation follows. Nurses' duty of care and the legal issues surrounding registration are then explored. The importance of continuing professional development is highlighted and devices such as profiles, reflection and accreditation of prior learning are introduced. The contribution of individualised care, primary nursing and nursing development units is evaluated. The potential of nursing models to identify and consolidate the unique contribution of nursing in care home settings is explored. Strategies for maximising teamwork are offered. Health and health promotion are considered in the context of older people. Equal opportunities and cultural sensitivity are supported as being fundamental to quality continuing care. Finally, suggestions regarding the successful management of change are offered.

Quality

Quality is an abstract concept which is difficult to define. Quality continuing care should satisfy residents'/clients' needs appropriately and effectively. Care should be fair, accessible and acceptable to the client group for which it has been provided (Maxwell, 1984). Measurements of quality concern the goodness of any technical care that is given, the goodness of the interpersonal relationship through which care is given and the goodness of the environment in which the care takes place (Donabedian, 1989). Quality must be the concern of everyone.

A Strategy for Nursing (DoH, 1989) outlines goals for standard setting, quality assessment and quality assurance. Quality assurance literally means to guarantee quality care, and standards which can be assessed and measured are fundamental to this process. Standards articulate an agreed level of care against which quality can be judged through the use of audit. The Dynamic Standard Setting System (DySSSy) developed by the Royal College of Nursing's Standards of Care Project (Royal College of Nursing, 1990) outlines three phases in the quality assurance cycle: describing and setting objectives, measuring and monitoring those objectives and taking action on the findings. The DySSSy system also advocates a 'bottom up' rather than 'top down' approach to quality assurance where all staff, including support staff, are involved in all stages of the quality assurance process. Audit involves monitoring standards to establish whether or not they are being met. This can be done through examining documentation, observing practice, individual/group reflection, and interviews and/or questionnaires with residents/clients and their relatives.

UKCC and National Boards

The 1979 Nurses, Midwives and Health Visitors Act established the United Kingdom Central Council (UKCC) and the four National Boards (Scotland, Northern Ireland, England and Wales) to regulate the nursing, midwifery and health visiting professions. One of the UKCC's main functions is to establish and improve standards of professional conduct. The title 'registered nurse' is legally protected and practising nurses have to be registered with the UKCC (Pyne, 1992).

The UKCC determines the standards required for entry to professional education and the kind, content and standard of that education. It decides when an individual should gain or lose the right to practise and is charged with protecting and improving standards of education and practice in the public interest. The UKCC consequently provides advice to all practitioners regarding the expected standards of professional conduct.

Nurses are responsible for ensuring that their practice is in line with the standards of the UKCC, which in turn is responsible to society for upholding the standards of the profession. Registered nurses are accountable for their practice. And this accountability applies at all times whether on or off duty and even when not employed as a nurse, for example if a nurse is working in a residential home (UKCC, 1989). Nurses are accountable not only for what they do but also what they do not do. For example, not giving prescribed medication is as much of a problem as giving the wrong medicine or getting the dose wrong.

So what is accountability?

The words responsibility and accountability are frequently taken to mean the same thing, and sometimes seem to be used almost interchangeably, but there is a difference. Being accountable means being answerable for actions or decisions to someone recognised as having the right to demand information and an explanation. Thus, through accepting registration, nurses are accountable to the UKCC for their professional actions; by accepting a job, nurses can be held to account by their employers and by accepting responsibility for clinical care, nurses can be held to account by residents/clients.

Responsibility is related to, but not the same as, accountability. Responsibility can be delegated to someone else, but accountability cannot. Accountability is *to* someone whereas responsibility is *for* someone or something (McNulty, 1980). For example nurses might delegate the total care needs of a resident in a nursing home to a care assistant, but they remain accountable for the standard of that same care and the appropriateness of that delegation.

Nurses must also acknowledge the limitations of their knowledge, skills and competence, and decline to perform those activities for which they have not been prepared (UKCC, 1992a, b). After initial registration, nurses must confirm their ability to practise every three years (UKCC, 1995). Registration therefore indicates that a certain level of knowledge and skill has been reached and that patients/clients can be assured of safe, professional care. Doctors, dentists and some other health care professionals have similar regulatory bodies.

Are student nurses accountable?

Increasingly student nurses are working in nursing homes and other continuing care settings as part of their clinical experience. Miller (1990) suggests that although student nurses can be held responsible for their actions, they are not professionally accountable. Accountability is achieved through the authority to practice which derives from the conferment of registration. Students cannot be accountable as they do not have the authority to make decisions, and must be always working under the supervision and guidance of a registered nurse. However, as Darbyshire (1989) points out, if a student assaults a resident/client while giving care, it is not really feasible to say that the college of nursing is at fault because it did not prepare the student adequately for the stresses and strains of clinical work, or that it is the registered nurse's fault because she did not physically stand over and supervise the student at all times and therefore prevent such an assault happening.

In addition, we are all as citizens accountable to the law and all have a common law 'duty of care'. Nurses and student nurses can therefore be challenged to account for their actions or omissions in court. The code of professional conduct in itself does not have legal force, but breach of the code can be used in evidence against a party in a court action (Dimond, 1991).

Nurses are accountable to residents/clients for the delivery of care of a high standard which is effective, safe and ethically good. The needs of the residents/clients are paramount and predominate over those of the practitioner and the profession. Residents and clients are increasingly more able to objectively evaluate their care in an informed manner, as a result of improved general education standards and the media coverage particularly on television of health care matters. Similarly the Patient's Charter (DoH, 1991) embodies a changed view of resident/client rights and ways of satisfying them. Public trust and confidence in nursing is dependent on its practitioners being seen to exercise their accountability responsibly. Nursing is a self-regulating profession which means that nurses are accountable to other nurses and judged against criteria set by nurses.

Nurses must also work collaboratively and co-operatively with other professionals, and recognise and respect their particular contributions to care. Nurses are accountable to their multi-disciplinary colleagues for carrying out their plans and providing them with feedback. Nurses are accountable to their employer for providing the service which they are employed to provide, for the proper use of resources and conforming to locally devised policy. If nurses do not feel competent to carry out a particular aspect of care they must ensure that they negotiate access to the required training and supervision to be able to carry out that skill safely.

If a nurse believes that a resident or client in their care is not progressing as he or she ought to, the nurse has a duty to record this in the notes and to inform the relevant people. Sometimes nurses feel reluctant to do this as they fear it may be taken by others to indicate that they are not coping or are incompetent. However, not reporting a deterioration shows a lack of professionalism and more importantly demonstrates a lack of concern for the well-being of the resident/client (Watson, 1992).

Similarly nurses are accountable for their professional judgements about treatment: whether or not this was the correct course of action for the particular individual as well as the cost-effectiveness of the treatment implemented and the resources used. Consequently nurses must be aware of current thinking and research. Personal preference, for example, just liking one type of dressing better than another, is not a sufficient basis for recommendation. Neither is tradition or 'we've always done it this way'. There are, however, often no simple answers to many nursing problems. For example, an emergency situation may require immediate action and there may be no precedent for the event which has occurred. In such cases the nurse must act instinctively and do her best – after all this is what being an autonomous professional is all about (Tingle, 1990).

In order to be accountable, what do nurses need?

To be accountable nurses must see themselves as having a clearly defined role with its own skills, knowledge base, aims and research objectives and understand that this role entails specific and distinct responsibilities which belong to nobody else (Hunt, 1991). To be accountable therefore nurses should be able not only to give the care that is required, but also to explain why it was given in the way it was. Consequently nurses need appropriate up-to-date, research-based knowledge and the authority to act with a reasonable degree of autonomy. Nurses must be capable of independent thought and committed to the idea of continuing professional education and development.

The Scope of Professional Practice

In the past, as a result of guidance from the Department of Health in 1977, if nurses wanted to take on duties or responsibilities that were not usually associated with the nurse's role or covered in pre-registration education, such as intravenous drug administration or suturing, employers would demand further locally-based training. Consequently if nurses changed employer they often had to do the new employer's course even if they had done another one elsewhere very recently. This led to much unnecessary duplication and professional frustration, and was extremely wasteful of resources. However, the UKCC launched a liberating document entitled 'The scope of professional practice' in 1992 which put the responsibility for competence in such roles and duties firmly on the individual nurse. Nurses are now expected to acknowledge any limitations of knowledge, skill and competence and take steps to remedy them. In this respect nurses are free to exercise their own judgement as to the tasks they take on as long as any new role adopted does not adversely affect patient care or put them outside the Code of Professional Conduct.

Advocacy and whistleblowing

All practitioners who are registered on the UKCC's register are required to set and achieve high standards. Advocacy on the behalf of residents/clients therefore is an essential feature of the exercise of accountability by nurses. However, the nurse must use her professional judgement as to how and when to advocate. In many situations there may well be a tension between the maintenance of standards and the availability or use of resources. Even though it may seem much more straightforward and simple to 'look the other way', this could be seen as contrary to professional behaviour and the nurse could be called to account. '… Blind, unthinking, unquestioning obedience, refusing to challenge anything …' is unacceptable as it will frequently expose residents/clients to risks (Pyne, 1992). Fear of disapproval is no excuse for keeping quiet.

The Code of Professional Conduct (UKCC, 1992a) applies to all persons on the register regardless of the post held. It is intended to be a support to practitioners who are concerned about standards of care. However, complaining about standards of care, or 'whistleblowing' is fraught with difficulties. If nurses express concern at the situations which lead to poor care they may risk censure from their employers. On the other hand, however, if they do not make their concerns known, they are then vulnerable to complaint from the UKCC for failing to justify its standards and their registration may be in jeopardy. Nurses who choose to 'whistle-blow' are also faced with a difficult balancing act concerning whether or not to reveal matters about patient care which are in the public interest against maintaining patient confidentiality and public confidence in the service.

For many older people, the care staff are their sole advocates. Should nurses decide to take action regarding poor standards of care, an essential part of the process is accurate record-keeping. Records should be completed at the time of the incident or problem and should detail the consequences for the residents/clients who have not been given the care they needed and deserved. Any deficit in the care given to an individual patient/client should be recorded in their nursing notes and a formal report made to the manager of the care area. Copies should be sent to the nurse's local professional organisation or union representative. The situation should also be discussed with the professional staff of the UKCC. If the nurse feels unable to complain to her line manager she should side-step them and go to the top.

Making a complaint is never going to be an easy thing to do as it involves the difficult decision of balancing the potential personal, financial and professional costs against doing what is right. The protection of membership of a trade union and/or professional organisation is crucial. Whatever happens, going to the press should only be the very last resort. Many employers now include clauses in their contracts of employment forbidding employees to speak to the press or outside bodies.

Legal issues

All nursing activities carry legal implications as nurses owe a legal duty of care to their patients (Tingle, 1992). Every nursing activity carries the potential for a charge of negligence.

Negligence can also result from mismanagement, wrongful delegation, failure to observe residents/clients and so on. If a resident/client suffers harm from a nurse's actions or omissions they could be personally sued by that resident/client. The law fortunately does not expect nurses to be superhuman. If a negligence case was brought to court, the nurse's actions would be judged against what could have been expected from an ordinarily skilled nurse in the same speciality. Not the very best, most perfect nurse, but an ordinary one. Nevertheless nurses should make sure they are up-to-date, skilled and knowledgeable.

Research-based practice

There is still a belief that time spent away from practice, reading in the library or attending study days, is not real work. A Strategy for Nursing (DoH, 1989) has as one of its key aims an intention to promote research-based practice. Research is a scientific, systematic approach to gaining knowledge or understanding. Justification for the importance of applying research findings to practice commonly centres on four main factors: improving patient care; the professionalisation of nursing, enhancing accountability and promoting cost-effective care (Bircumshaw, 1990). If research findings are to be used in practice, then dissemination is absolutely crucial. The establishment of a journal club, where members share the responsibility of keeping each other up-to-date, can be extremely beneficial.

Continuing professional development

In the past, students of nursing learned on an apprenticeship type model where learning the basic technical skills of the job was seen as the priority. Educational needs came second to service needs with clinical placements and study leave being to a large extent dictated by service requirements rather than the needs and learning objectives of the student.

Project 2000 – a new preparation for practice (UKCC, 1986) heralded a far reaching change. Students have supernumerary status, that is, they are not counted in the numbers, and students of all branches of nursing share the first 18 months of their education. The theoretical content is derived from the disciplines of nursing, health, sociology, psychology, physiology, social policy, law and ethics and is founded on concepts of health rather than illness. Students are also expected to be research minded and computer literate. Students work in both institutional and non-institutional settings, receive a higher education diploma on qualification, and undergo a period of preceptorship or supported professional development once qualified. Increasingly significant numbers of the clinical placements are provided by the independent and voluntary sectors.

Profiles

The UKCC has made it a requirement for re-registration after April 1998, that nurses must be involved in continuing professional development – a minimum of five days (or equivalent) over three years – and that they maintain a professional profile (UKCC, 1995). The profile should contain evidence which demonstrates the continuing acquisition of skills, knowledge, attitudes, understanding and achievement.

The UKCC has established five broad areas for development: patient, client and colleague support; care enhancement; practice development; reducing risk, and education development. Evidence of learning acquired from reflection on everyday practice experience is also required.

From April 2000, if nurses have had a break in practice, that is, if they have worked less than 100 days or 750 hours in the previous five years, they will be required to complete a statutory Return to Practice programme and to demonstrate that they are able to provide safe and competent care before renewing their registration. All return to practice programmes must be approved by the relevant National Board.

Reflection

Reflection is a term used to refer to personal exploration of experiences in order to lead to new understanding and learning (Boud et al., 1985). Many authors argue that reflection improves practice. It is suggested that writing about experiences allows nurses to review experiences more deeply and to learn from them more effectively. Some people use a reflective diary on a regular basis to record specific events. Others use reflective journals to review their learning and development over a longer period of time. Particular benefits can be gained by sharing reflections with a colleague or mentor.

(For details about further study, APL, APEL and CATS see Chapter 9).

Clinical nurse specialists

Historically, nurses wishing to advance their careers had to choose between education and management. However, a need for specialist practitioners to remain at the 'bedside' in order to promote and enhance innovations in care has been acknowledged (UKCC, 1995). All specialist practitioners will have to demonstrate achievement in relation to clinical practice, leadership, practice development and care and programme management. To obtain a specialist practitioner qualification, nurses will need to undertake a programme of education to a standard set by the UKCC and approved by the appropriate National Board which will be at least at first-degree level. The Clinical Nurse Specialist role, with its emphasis on expert knowledge, research, education and practice skills, would appear an ideal mechanism for developing nursing practice within continuing care settings.

Individualised care, primary nursing and nursing development units

The nursing process was developed initially for educational purposes in the USA in the 1950s, and adopted into practice in the UK in the 1970s. It aimed to provide better nursing care by means of a systematic, individualised approach. These initiatives formed part of a drive to counteract falling standards of care and low morale due to the 'production-line', mechanistic and depersonalising concept of task-focused care. Within the nursing process, the patient was promoted as being at the centre of the care process, nurses were urged to give total patient care and values such as holism and individuality were emphasised.

Primary Nursing

Primary nursing was developed in the USA by Marie Manthey in the 1960s as a more effective method of organising nursing care delivery. It emphasises the allocation and acceptance of accountability and responsibility for decision-making (and the majority of care-giving) about a small group of patients to one nurse from admission to discharge. On its introduction to the UK in the early 1980s certain philosophical attributes were also stressed such as the importance of viewing the patient as a whole, the need for partnership between patient and nurse, and the therapeutic role of the nurse–patient relationship in the care process. The value and uniqueness of the individual was also highlighted (Black, 1992). A central feature of primary nursing was a belief that the nurse–patient relationship is therapeutic and beneficial in its own right. The need to give residents/clients more control and choice over care is emphasised (Wright, 1986; Pearson, 1988).

Primary nursing carries with it major implications in terms of responsibility, accountability and competence. The allocation and acceptance of responsibility for decision-making to one individual is perhaps the most important difference between primary nursing and other more traditional systems of care such as task allocation. In primary nursing, primary nurses have their own case-loads and the care-giver on one shift reports directly to the care-giver coming on duty, communicates with other members of the care team and with the resident/client and their family.

Nursing Development Units

Nursing Development Units (NDUs) emerged in the early 1980s as places to foster and encourage the development of nurses and nursing through promoting innovation in practice. Four were created with assistance from the King's Fund in 1989, and a Government grant supported another thirty from 1992–1995. Networking and other small grants have encouraged many others to develop. NDUs, however established and funded, focus on the development of advanced nursing practice where experimentation in therapeutic and patient-centred nursing care is encouraged, facilitated and supported (Lathlean and Vaughan, 1994). Change and creativity are accepted as the norm and NDUs provide settings where innovations such as complementary therapies, nursing models, and alternative ways of managing and organising care can be developed and tested. NDUs need to be supported by good education, management and research and are committed to sharing the insights gained with others.

Nursing as therapy

Old age has traditionally been seen in many health care settings as an illness which advances progressively and irreversibly towards death. This bio-medical model offers a rather passive and merely palliative role for nurses. Although 'good nursing care' within this model can compensate for many of the common consequences of old age such as impaired mobility, incontinence and dementia, the adoption of a broader model of care has much more to offer nurses. There is a need to develop and measure the enormous therapeutic potential of nursing. For example, there has recently been a proliferation of techniques such as reality orientation, reminiscence therapy, biography, life review, aromatherapy, massage and therapeutic touch which some nurses have incorporated into their practice. The direct therapeutic relevance of such approaches has been questioned by some authors; nevertheless continuing care settings would appear to provide an excellent milieu for the implementation and rigorous evaluation of such therapies.

Nursing models

Doreen Norton saw the continuing care of older people as representing true nursing. The curative bio-medical model of care which dominates in acute health care settings is inappropriate in continuing care as it prevents nursing from developing fully its therapeutic potential. Nursing models are descriptions of nursing and the ideas and areas of interest to nursing. They are intended to clarify thinking about the purpose of nursing, and the knowledge needed for practice. Continuing care requires a different, but well-grounded, theoretical approach. Nursing models need to be adopted to make explicit nursing's therapeutic function, and support a positive approach to the health promotion of older people in continuing care settings. All nursing models deal with four essential concepts, namely person, environment, health and the nature of nursing.

Person

Nursing models include ideas about the nature of people who require care. The most consistent idea is that of wholeness or holism; that is, that the person is greater than the sum of his parts and therefore that the person cannot be reduced to his constituent parts without losing something in the process.

Health

Health is usually identified as the purpose or goal of nursing. Some models use ideas of a health–illness continuum with the nurse's purpose being to assist the person to achieve the highest degree of health possible. Others view health as something more, or different from, the absence of disease, that is, as a dynamic changing life process. Many view health as being interdependent with the environment and others view it as something within the individual.

Environment

The environment in which care is carried out is perceived as being essential to nursing but is often not examined as fully as the other concepts. Several theorists view the environment as a critical interacting force shaping the individual. For example Nightingale saw the primary focus for nursing as altering the physical environment so as to place the person for the healing processes of nature to work.

The nature of nursing

Nursing is generally viewed as a helping process with a primary focus on interpersonal interactions. This helps identify the knowledge and skills needed for nursing practice. Theorists offer alternative perspectives on who controls the process of nursing; that is, whether the patient/client controls and the nurse facilitates and enables or that the control is equally shared or even totally initiated by the nurse.

Why we need models?

In the past nurses tended to base their practice on intuition, experience or 'the way it has always been done'. Leddy and Pepper (1993) argue that such approaches led to routine and stereotyped practice. Much of present knowledge about practice remains limited. For example, little is known and articulated about when and why nursing is successful, and what it is nurses do that makes a difference. There is now, however, increasing pressure on nurses, from educationalists, managers and academics, to base their practice on theory.

Nursing models help nurses to challenge existing practices and provide different ways to think about problems. Nursing models help nurses focus on nursing rather than medical issues. They encourage nurses to explore the diversity of health rather than purely the pathology and focus on the whole person and their 'significant others' rather than simply their body parts. Nursing models offer guidelines for practice. They help nurses identify which problems nursing can solve and what the goal of nursing ought to be. Models also offer a framework for assessment, intervention and evaluation, thereby assisting nurses in analysing their practice and giving direction to the goals of nursing care. Finally, models identify who should be carrying out nursing activities. This appears a particularly relevant and useful function in the context of today's dilemmas concerning skill mix and expanded roles.

Health promotion

The World Health Organisation declaration at Alma Ata in 1978 advocated a key role for nurses in health promotion. Health promotion roles and activities are diverse in continuing care settings and should include: restoring and maintaining health and independence and enabling older people with disabilities (whether physical or mental) to achieve their fullest potential and ensuring death with dignity. In addition, because nurses spend more continuous time with older people in their care, they have a valuable role in the early recognition of significant changes that may require intervention from other professionals. Health is, however, extremely difficult to define.

Dimensions of health

Ewles and Simnett (1995) have isolated six dimensions of health: physical, mental, emotional, social, spiritual and societal that are useful in helping to understand this elusive concept more fully.

- Physical health is concerned with optimal mechanical functioning of the body.
- Mental health involves maintaining the ability to think clearly and coherently.
- Emotional health includes recognising and expressing emotions appropriately.
- Social health highlights the importance of making and maintaining relationships.
- Spiritual health requires support of the individual's religious or personal philosophy on life.
- Societal health encourages a broader look at society and social issues in general such as the need to promote equal opportunities, lobby for anti-ageist policies and have a concern for the environment.

Intervention aimed at addressing each of these six dimensions is vital in developing a health promoting approach to care in continuing care areas.

Multi-professional working

The varied needs of many older people often leads to the simultaneous involvement of a number of agencies and professional groups. Effective team work is important and necessary to ensure that contributions from some disciplines do not become submerged and ignored. It is important to ensure that accurate assessments are carried out and appropriate referrals made. For this approach to be successful, there should be regular communication and sharing of ideas. Long- and short-term goals should be set, and each discipline should monitor its own input. There should be a clear understanding by each team member of the role, function, skills and responsibilities of the other team members.

Equal opportunities and culturally sensitive care

The NHS and Community Care Act (1990) emphasises that people from different cultural backgrounds may have different care needs. Immigration to Britain (mainly since the 1950s) has meant that significant numbers of older people from minority ethnic groups will need continuing care. Little is known about the actual health needs and continuing care expectations of black and ethnic minority communities. Care provision must be acceptable and appropriate to be effective.

Stewart (1991) points out that:

> If I say 'the British eat fish and chips' you would doubtless agree that this is a correct assumption. The reality is that 25 per cent of the population do so on a regular basis, therefore what is seen as a British tradition is in fact untrue for 75 per cent of the people.

Understanding of, and provision for, cultural differences is crucial. A colour blind service may appear to offer 'equality' but, where take-up is disproportionate, questions must be asked of appropriateness, awareness, access and acceptability.

Equal opportunities is concerned with eliminating discrimination on grounds of sex, race, age and marital status. The black communities in the UK have played a major part in the building and maintenance of health care provision. However, they continue to be concentrated in unskilled, low-status and poorly-paid positions (King's Fund, 1990). Positive strategies for change include the wider use of ethnic monitoring, the destruction of racist stereotypes, and positive action in terms of recruitment. Education of staff at all levels is essential, and input from older people themselves helps dispel myths and stereotypes.

Managing change

Change is a fundamental part of life as a professional. The pitfalls associated in the change process have long been recognised. For example, in 1513, Machiavelli identified that:

> There is nothing more difficult to carry out, nor more dangerous to handle, than to initiate a new order of things. For the reformer has enemies in all who profit by the old order, and only lukewarm defenders in all who profit by the new order. The lukewarmness arises partly from fear of their adversaries, who have law in their favour, and partly from the incredulity of mankind who do not truly believe in anything new until they have had actual experience of it.

Many changes fail because of a lack of planning and strategy. All change will meet with some resistance and resistance often springs from fear. However, it is also important to acknowledge that resistance may be a useful warning to reassess aims and objectives thus leading to a new plan. Therefore it is important to involve as many of those affected as possible in all stages of the change process, to keep channels of communication open, to be prepared to negotiate and to evaluate constantly.

Resistance can also be minimised by planning the change process carefully, identifying potential problems before they happen, and carefully considering all alternatives. Much of the role of the nurse in continuing care settings is to facilitate planned change. To carry out this role nurses require certain skills such as social awareness, good interpersonal skills, power, resilience, persistence and flexibility.

Change is more likely to succeed if there is openness, good interpersonal and informational links, freedom from organisational constraints, supportive leadership and trust (ENB, 1987).

Conclusion

Nursing older people in continuing care settings is an extremely complex activity, requiring advanced knowledge and expert practice skills. This chapter provided an overview of key professional issues that are fundamental to the development of nursing in continuing care. Expectations of professional nursing practice with regard to quality of care and accountability have been outlined. The centrality of continuing professional development was stressed. Individualised care, primary nursing and nursing development units have been highlighted as ways of developing practice and the therapeutic potential of nursing in continuing care settings. Nursing models have been advocated in place of the more restrictive bio-medical model as a foundation for practice, and health promotion has been suggested as a legitimate goal for care. Finally the importance of equal opportunities and cultural sensitivity was defended and strategies for managing change were summarised.

Useful Contacts

Commission for Racial Equality, Elliot House, 10–12 Allington Street, London SW1E 5EH. Tel: 0171 828 7022.

RCN Whistleblow, Freepost 23, London W1E 2XX.

UKCC, 23 Portland Place, London W1N 3AF. Tel: 0171 637 7181. Fax: 0171 436 2924.

References

Bircumshaw, D. (1990) the utilisation of research findings in clinical nursing practice. *Journal of Advanced Nursing*, **15**, 1272–1280.
Black, F. (ed.) (1992) *Primary Nursing: an Introductory Guide*. London: King's Fund.
Boud, D., Keogh, R. and Walker, D. (1985) *Reflection: Turning Experience into Learning*. London, Kogan Page.
Darbyshire, P. (1989) Responsibility, accountability and advocacy: student nurse dilemmas. Part II. *Irish Nursing Forum and Health Services*, May/June, 18–20.
Department of Health (1989) A Strategy for Nursing. London: DoH.
Department of Health (1991) The Patient's Charter. London: HMSO.
Department of Health (1990) The NHS and Community Care Act. London: HMSO.

Dimond, B. (1991) All part of the job. *Nursing Times*, **87**, 33, 44–46.

Donabedian, A. (1989) Institutional and professional responsibilities in quality assurance. *Quality Assurance in Health Care*, **1**(1) 3–11.

ENB (1987) Managing change in nursing education. Pack I: Preparing for change. London: English National Board for Nursing, Midwifery and Health Visiting.

ENB (1989) Managing change in nursing education. Pack II: Workshop materials for action. London: English National Board for Nursing, Midwifery and Health Visiting.

ENB (1992) Framework for continuing professional education. London: English National Board for Nursing, Midwifery and Health Visiting.

Evans, A. (1993) Accountability a core concept for primary nursing. *Journal of Clinical Nursing*, **2**, 231–234.

Ewles, L. and Simnett, I. (1995) *Promoting Health: A Practical Guide* (3rd edition). London: Scutari Publications Ltd.

Gardner, J.H. (1992) Where the buck stops. *Nursing*, **5**, 3, 14–16

Hunt, G. (1991) Professional accountability. *Nursing Standard*, **6**, 4, 49–50.

Keighley, T. (1989) Developments in quality assurance. *Senior Nurse*, **9**(9), 7–10.

King Edward's Hospital Fund for London (1990) Racial equality: the nursing profession. Equal Opportunities Task Force Occasional Paper, Number 6. London: King's Fund.

Lathlean, J. and Vaughan, B. (1994) *Unifying Nursing Practice and Theory*. Oxford: Butterworth-Heinemann.

Leddy, S. and Pepper, J.M. (1993) *Conceptual Bases of Professional Nursing*. Philadelphia: J. B. Lippincott.

Maxwell, R.J. (1984) Quality assessment in health. *British Medical Journal*, **288**, 1470–1472.

McNulty, B. (1980) *Accountability Shared with Other Professions*. London: Royal College of Nursing.

Miller, J. (1990) Registration makes a nurse accountable. *Nursing Times*, **86**, 27.

Pyne, R. (1992) Breaking the code. *Nursing*, **5**, 3, 8–10.

Royal College of Nursing (1990) *Quality Patient Care: The Dynamic Standard Setting System*. London: Royal College of Nursing.

Stewart, L. (1991) The way forward: education. In A.J. Squires (ed.) *Multicultural Health Care and Rehabilitation of Older People*, pp. 195–200. London: Edward Arnold.

Tingle, J. (1990) Ethics in practice. *Nursing Times*, **86**, 48, 54–55.

Tingle, J. (1992) Primary nursing and the law. *British Journal of Nursing*, **1**(5) 248–251.

UKCC (1986) Project 2000 – a new preparation for practice.

UKCC (1989) Exercising accountability. London: United Kingdom Central Council for Nursing, Midwifery and Health Visiting.

UKCC (1992a) The Code of Professional Conduct (3rd edition). London: United Kingdom Central Council for Nursing, Midwifery and Health Visiting.

UKCC (1992b) The Scope of Professional Practice. London: United Kingdom Central Council for Nursing, Midwifery and Health Visiting.

UKCC (1995) PREP and you: maintaining your registration, standards for education following registration. London, United Kingdom Central Council for Nursing, Midwifery and Health Visiting.

Watson, R. (1992) Justifying your practice. *Nursing*, **5**, 3, 11–13.

Further Reading

Department of Health (1989) A Strategy for Nursing. London: Department of Health.

Department of Health (1991) The Patient's Charter. London: HMSO.

ENB (1992) Framework for continuing professional education. London: English National Board for Nursing, Midwifery and Health Visiting.

Royal College of Nursing (1990) Quality patient care: the dynamic standard setting system. London: RCN.

UKCC (1989) Exercising accountability. London: United Kingdom Central Council for Nursing, Midwifery and Health Visiting.

UKCC (1992a) The code of professional conduct. (3rd edition) London: United Kingdom Central Council for Nursing, Midwifery and Health Visiting.

UKCC (1992b) The scope of professional practice. London: United Kingdom Central Council for Nursing, Midwifery and Health Visiting.

UKCC (1995) PREP and you: maintaining your registration, standards for education following registration. London, United Kingdom Central Council for Nursing, Midwifery and Health Visiting.

4

What Older People Value in Nurses

Pauline Ford

Introduction

Nurses are key providers of health and social care and as such their work has come under increasing scrutiny by policy makers as well as service purchasers and providers in terms of cost-effectiveness and quality of service. In the present climate of cost-driven health services, nursing, more than ever before, must demonstrate its cost-effectiveness and its value. The change in culture has created a change for the consumers also. Consumer demands, consumer satisfaction and consumer involvement are terms which drop from everybody's lips. Even the Patient's Charter (DoH, 1991) exhorts us to ensure that the patient is put first and that services reflect the stated preferences of the consumer. Whatever the successes of community care, it has been asserted that some form of care home provision will always be needed (Henwood, 1992). It seems important therefore to establish the thoughts and views of those older people who are in receipt of continuing care services.

This chapter will explore such views through a review of the relevant literature and an original research study.

The value of nursing

Several studies have attempted to demonstrate the value of nursing. In 1991 Buchan and Ball reviewed British and American research which showed the benefits of employing qualified nurses. Studies by Bagust and Slack (1991), Bagust et al. (1992), and the University of York (1992), indicate that quality of care is dependent on using qualified nurses. The Audit Commission (1991) referred to the value and importance of qualified nurses in its report 'The Virtue of Patients'. All of these studies pointed to the relationship between the employment of qualified registered nurses and the provision of cost-effective quality care. To accompany the statistics on cost-effectiveness, the Royal College of Nursing published *The Value of Nursing* (1992), a qualitative record of real life experiences of nurses whose care had made a difference to patients. Since then, nurses who work with older people have produced *The Value and Skills of Nurses working with Older People*, (RCN, 1993b) and *Older People and Contining Care; the skill and value of the nurse* (RCN 1993a). Both of these publications attempt to articulate the value of nurses' work with older people and serve to assist the nurse in making the case for their continuing involvement in the provision of health and social care services for older people. The major focus of all this work has been on nursing and nurses. What is missing, however, is the perception of the user of the service.

Consumerism

If the experiences of older people and their degree of satisfaction goes some way to determining the quality of care, then obtaining those views must be a significant factor in the measurement of services for that client group. In reviewing the literature, it becomes clear that few of the studies on patient satisfaction have involved older people.

What then do older people want from nurses? In their review of the literature, Jones et al. (1987) indicated that staff–patient communication was the concern most frequently raised by patients, in relation to most health care professionals. They concluded that patients regarded easy exchange of thoughts and ideas as an essential part of therapy. Cornwell (1989) reported that older people seemed to feel more intensely than most the need for information. She refers to the important effect which the attitudes of health professionals have on users of the service, as frequently demonstrated by comments from patient and consumer organisations. Older people appear to feel especially strongly about professional attitudes and have indicated a strong need to be treated as individuals and with respect. Relationships with staff were identified as being of crucial importance.

Nurse led units

Excellent nursing homes have also been distinguished from ordinary nursing homes by the personal attention staff pay to residents (Anderson, 1987). Clark and Bowling (1989) found that the distinguishing feature of excellence were those homes which emphasised a rehabilitative rather than a custodial model of care. Rehabilitation nursing reflects a more participative approach to care which implies involvement of the client in establishing goals which reflect to some degree their needs and wants. Ebrahim (1993) drew attention to the value of a service which reflected clients' needs, promoting a sense of involvement in the day to day running of the establishment. It is, according to Ebrahim, the staff who 'make or break' the residents' quality of life in care settings. He argues that without any training or supervision it is inevitable that processes of care will adapt to suit staff rather than the residents.

The case for nurse-managed NHS nursing homes has been strongly advocated by nurses, (Wade et al., 1983; Baker, 1983) and by some doctors, (Batchelor, 1984). Three NHS nursing homes, headed by nurses, were established and demonstrated greater personal well-being for residents, higher consumer satisfaction and no increase in cost (Bond, 1984; Bond and Bond, 1987; Bond et al., 1989a, b). Clark and Bowling (1989), in a study comparing quality of life in two NHS nursing homes and one long-stay ward, concluded that quality of life was more positive in the homes. Pembry (1984) has argued that registered nurses are often not valued because because few opportunities exist to demonstrate that competent and professional nursing is beneficial to patients, is cost effective and that the nurse–patient relationship is in itself therapeutic. Raphael (1965) conducted a survey to compare the views of patients with those who cared for them, many patients expressed pleasure at being asked to give their views. She found that there was a strong, highly significant relationship between age and the satisfaction ratios expressed by patients. The older the patient the more contented they were. It has long been of interest to researchers and providers of health and social care services why this should be so. Furthermore Peace et al. (1979) and Willcocks et al. (1984) refer to the low expectation older people tend to have regarding institutional care. Associated with this inability or reluctance to offer critical evaluation, is the difficulty some older patients may experience in exercising consumer choice.

Contemplating greater involvement of older people in developing the nursing services they desire will inevitably have some bearing on the relationships currently experienced by nurses and patients.

Patient–nurse Relationships.

There is no shortage of literature on the subject of nurse–patient relationships, (see for example, Elander, 1993; Oliver and Redfern, 1992; Loveredge and Heineken, 1988; Meutzal, 1988). There is, however, less published work on patients' perceptions of the relationship between patients and nurses.

Huss et al. (1988) explored the relationship between residents in long-term care, nursing staff and the association of such relationships to residents' life satisfaction. Thirty residents were interviewed using various indexes, such as the nurse–resident relationship tool, adapted from an instrument developed by Risser (1975), in order to evaluate patient satisfaction with nurses and nursing care. Results indicated a significantly higher life satisfaction score for patients who reported having a 'confidant'. This result is consistent with findings reported by Lowenthal and Haven (1976) which suggested that individuals who have 'confidants' exhibit higher morale. The correlation between life satisfaction and the nurse–patient relationship was not statistically significant. Nurses contributed to this only through their roles as 'confidant'. This would appear to suggest (at least for those patients participating in this study) that nurses should have a close interpersonal relationship with their clients to be effective in contributing to the life satisfaction of their patients. In an interesting social network analysis, Powers (1992) studied the different ways in which health care residents interpret their relationships with

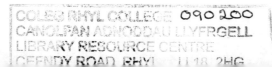

staff. The study took place in an American, state-operated long-term care establishment, between 1984 and 1986. Patients were aged 55 years and over. This study identified that patients who

> ... had lost or become distanced from their highly supportive people in their pre-institution networks ... were more apt to turn toward staff as a source of dependent support and emotional attachment ...

There is evidence to suggest that some networks may evolve in response to changes across an individual's lifespan, for example, due to geographic relocation or the death of important network members (Wenger, 1989). Powers (1992) recommends longitudinal study to aid the understanding of older people's social networks. In her study she concludes that:

> In long term care, appreciating and learning to use informal personal relationships to maintain communication between staff and residents aids problem solving and may avert crisis.

It would seem that relationships in the context of health care are an important aspect of the experience of that care. Yet research on the perceptions of nurses and patients, as givers and receivers of care, elicits diverse and opposing views. Larson undertook a study which indicated that patients consistently value competent/knowledgeable actions to be more important than expressive behaviours, yet nurses were found to value expressive caring behaviours towards their patients (Larson, 1984). These findings have been confirmed by other studies, (see for example, Cronin and Harrison, 1988; Mangold, 1991; Von Essen and Sjoden, 1991; Rosenthal, 1992). Smith (1992) asked patients to describe a 'good nurse'. Utilising Coser's interview guide, her sample was drawn from a mixed age group of patients. Words used to describe nurses' functional skills included 'efficient, observant, alert and capable of doing their job'. The caring/emotional aspects of nursing were clearly seen as distinct but complementary to the functional aspects. Patients, when asked to describe their ideal nurse, used words such as 'kindness, helpfulness, patience, talking, listening, showing interest and sympathy'.

Relationships in continuing care settings

Thorne and Robinson (1989) argue that in many instances human interaction can represent the totality of what health care professionals have to offer. In their American ongoing 'Health Care Relationships' project they explore qualitatively what happens over time in the relationships that develop between chronically ill patients and health care providers from the perspective of the patient and family members involved.

Thorne and Robinson (1988) state that elder informants have aided understanding about the evolution of health care relationships for those with a chronic illness across the life span. Trends in the accounts shed light upon the unique aspects of older people's experiences, with shifting beliefs about health care relationships. Whilst this study is American and focuses in particular on relationships with doctors, it contains important information for nurses. The older people in this study valued hospitality, social interaction, reciprocity and expected their doctor to be more paternalistic than the younger informants did. It would be interesting to set up a similar study in this country, focusing on the value that older people place on nurses.

Peace (1993) cautions us about residents' perspectives on institutional life. There is evidence that certain aspects of life are important and valued. Despite this she states:

> ... that these findings, in many ways reflect the interests of researchers and the questions asked. When users set the questions the answers may be different.

Conclusions from the literature

The idea that patients themselves could and should take an active part in assessing quality of care was first endorsed by the Wagner Report, (Sinclair, 1988) and then in the White Paper Caring for People (1989) and the NHS and Community Care Act (DoH, 1990).

The active involvement of older people may assist professionals in achieving quality of life for consumers of continuing care services. The challenge is to find ways of overcoming the fears of those who still feel the expert should be in charge. The remainder of this chapter describes some of the findings from a study which attempted to ascertain the value which older people who are residents in continuing care settings, place on nursing. The study is valuable not only for its findings, but for the lessons learned about the processes of obtaining the views of older people.

The research process

The literature suggested that the views of older people should be treated with some caution because, perhaps more so than any other consumer group, they are eager to please. However, I was keen that older people should remain at the centre of my study and have control over the research process. To facilitate this I gathered the views of older people themselves about the process of the research. Discussions were held with patients both in groups and individually in order to obtain their views. Particularly valuable were their thoughts on the kinds of questions I should ask in order to elicit values, the language I was using, and my overall approach. Of particular concern was any interpretation of my motive for the study. Clearly if they felt I was undertaking a consumer satisfaction study, perhaps for management, then this would influence the findings. These people gave me clear, sound, common sense answers to my queries; enabling me to develop a relatively uncomplicated interview schedule for the actual research study.

The study was undertaken in a continuing care setting and involved interviewing the research participants individually, and also as members of a group. Throughout each stage of the process, my findings and plans for the next stage were discussed with, and validated by, the older people who were the research participants. Additionally I worked closely with a colleague who monitored my research process and of course with the research supervisor.

The findings of the study

The findings are described through direct quotes from the interview transcripts, which provide a framework for discussion. The participants' statements are written in italic font and, for clarity, the discussion is structured under three headings: The nurse, The patient and The nurse–patient relationship. The findings are not interpreted and this is purposeful, they are presented in such a way as to leave the reader to make his/her own interpretation. In this way the findings remain essentially individual; to the researcher, the research participants and to the reader. The findings are, however, related to those of other studies.

The nurse

Learning and assessing

The research participants identified student nurses as being novices, learning from qualified nurses and residents. A clear distinction of the good student was one who wanted to satisfy the patient, this was identified particularly through their interest in the individual needs of the patient.

> *I mean they've all got to learn, like we've had a student nurse here, Caroline, she left us last week, and she was getting to do the bandages, and she said to me, how I'm doing Stan? I said to her, you're doing a lovely job on them my love, well that pleased her, she wanted to do it.*

This nurse learnt by involving the patient in the learning process, giving pleasure to both the nurse and the patient. In their rush to 'assess' patients, nurses may forget that the patient is assessing them. This is demonstrated in Altschul's (1972) study which concluded that patients observe nurses and feel they know what nurses are like. For the older patient this assessment may take some time. Appearance, cleanliness, efficiency and kindness are some of the first things to be assessed. The older person then decides whether the nurse is a 'nice person', whether they will get on with each other and how competent the nurse is. There was a general view that newly qualified nurses had the ideal traits of a good nurse but were still learning. There was an acceptance of this need to learn as long as the patients were involved in the learning and the member of staff was a permanent appointment.

Intuition

When considering expert nurses the nurse would ideally have appropriate knowledge, skills and desired personal traits. These kinds of nurses were described as the real experts.

> *They do so much more with what they do know.*

Benner (1984) believes that one of the attributes of expert nurses is that they are intuitive. It is this attribute that the participants seemed to value particularly highly. It would seem that intuitive nurses are self aware, rendering them reflective and insightful.

> *She seems to know what you want almost before you know it yourself.*

The use of more personal and intuitive skills to supplement and build upon nursing knowledge can lead to a more reflective and intuitive approach to nursing. Rew and Barton (1989) point out that such an open minded and creative approach to care can lead to individualised nursing interventions. If more emphasis could be placed on outcomes of care then the 'expert' approach may receive more recognition. The nature of good professional nursing then seems to have several key elements: a sound knowledge base, perception and personality.

> *I want them to be understanding, knowledgeable and to know when I really need help.*

This implies that the nurse may need to reframe the patient's needs according to the knowledge and experience of the nurse, the individuality of the patient and the way the nurse feels about the resident's needs. The nature of the relationship between the nurse and the older person is crucial here. The nurse must recognise that it is the patient who has the clearest insight into their personal needs.

> *I want a nurse to know when I really need them, my needs are individual and a nurse really has to know what she is doing. They know a lot but they don't know it all.*

This was just one of many statements which indicates the individuality of patients' needs and their view that they have something to contribute. Expert nurses were described as insightful, professional and knowledgeable. The participants felt they deserved qualified nurses but went on to say,

> *It is a gift to be a good nurse.*

Whilst they felt they deserved qualified nurses, not all qualified nurses were considered to be good. It seemed that efficiency and personality made the difference. Nurses can be taught techniques to assist in promoting efficiency. However it is less clear whether the attributes of intuition, highly valued by the participants, can be developed through nurse training. To an extent it is likely that perceptiveness, if already present can be further developed thus rendering the expert nurse intuitive. But the question remains, are the qualities of the nurse intrinsic and part of personality? How much is learned or acquired through experience? Certainly a genuine interest in and liking of older people would be a requirement along with interpersonal and communication skills. But not all qualified nurses were considered to be good nurses and it appears that for the participants good nurses were also the ones who demonstrated that they cared.

Caring

> *Well its all in kindness, a nurse has got to be. S/he's got to have more than the job, s/he's got to be patient and kind to you. It's difficult to explain, it's compassion, really caring.*

A number of sociologists have attempted to define care (for example Graham, 1983; Ungerson, 1983a, b; 1990). Graham (1983) for example describes caring as both labour and love, caring for and caring about. To Benner and Wrubel (1989) caring is understanding the lived experience. They view the nurse as being with the patient in such a way as to try and share their humanity. Benner and Wrubel (1989) refer to this level of 'being with the patient' as 'presencing', a term used to try and capture the essence of truly being with and empathising with a patient. For Paterson and Zderad (1976) nursing is the nurturing response of one person to another in need. They urge the nurse to be with the patient in the fullest sense, the participants describe this as a sense of love.

> *A nurse has to be more than a nurse, … s/he has to have a lot of patience, understand you and be very loving. Some of the nurses are ever so loving and that's what you appreciate.*

For Paterson and Zderad (1976) nursing is viewed as a lived dialogue, involving the patient in the fullest sense of being open and available, being attentive and giving of self. Here I believe lies the key to the good nursing described in this study. The research participants were quite clear that any nurse working with them should be kind, caring and competent. The good nurse however was intuitive and gave a sense of being with the resident.

> *A nurse has to be more than a nurse … s/he has to have,…well s/he has to know what you need and what you want.*

Good nurses therefore demonstrate more than technical skill and kindness. Good nurses reach out and touch in a way which demonstrates genuine caring, making patients feel loved. This emphasis on caring and compassion can be allied to what Paterson and Zderad (1976) describe as the humanistic approach to nursing in which human interests, values and dignity are taken to be of primary importance. They suggest that the object of good nursing is to view the individual as a whole with emphasis on the individual's own perspective of the lived experience.

In order to achieve this, it could be argued that the nurse must approach nursing as an existential experience. In other words she must view nursing itself as a lived experience, a response to a human situation which the nurse shares with the patient. This kind of nursing is what I believe the participants meant by 'more than a nurse'. The nurse has to personally invest in being a good nurse, it cannot be superimposed.

> *My ideal nurse is intuitive, gives that little bit extra and goes beyond the call of duty. They are few in number and it depends greatly upon their personality. A nurse who really cares does things differently and they are greatly valued by the patients. It is the way things are done which makes the difference.*

True caring then appears to be based on an attitude of nurturing, of investing oneself in the experience of another sufficiently to be a participant in that person's experience. However, Smith (1992) argues that such levels of caring are devalued as a result of being seen as unsophisticated women's work. This is particularly evident in continuing care settings where the value of the qualified nurse's work is often unrecognised. It could be argued that this in turn marginalises care and attention to the 'little things'. Yet 'caring' is an important notion for the study's participants. It is demonstrated by attention to the 'little things'. (which matter to the patient.) For the research participants such attention to detail is seen as an essential ingredient of the expert nurse and such levels of caring appear to result in the nurse intuitively knowing the patient.

The resident

Loss and dependency

For the participants of this study, the ward is their home. Giving up their own homes was associated with loss of territory, loved ones and independence. This sense of loss appears exacerbated for those with no living relatives. Added to physical disability it places the individual in a highly dependent situation. Sixsmith (1986) suggests that dependency means three interrelated things to older people: not being able to do things for yourself, having to depend on others, and not being able to do what you want when you want. For the participants of this study it also meant having nowhere else to go. They all describe the challenge of being a continuing care patient in terms of accepting the loss of their homes. Home is now the ward where they live but its future is no more secure than hundreds of other continuing care wards which have been closed. The continuing care debate is inevitably affecting the research participants:

I sold my house because I was burgled and because I was told that I could stay here. Where will I go? I'll have to try and get a council house.

There had been no involvement of the participants in discussions with planners and policy makers regarding the future provision of continuing care. Feelings of powerlessness and distress were evident. They want to stay in their home.

Self-esteem

Dependency and feelings of powerlessness inevitably affect self-esteem which forms the foundation of psycho-social health and provides a measure for quality of life.

I'm absolutely dependent on these people, I can't do a thing myself.

The participants' self-esteem and sense of well-being is not enhanced by the frequent use of temporary staff and by the use of inexperienced staff.

I know they've got to learn but they should leave us somebody who is experienced. We deserve somebody who has experience.

Self-esteem is commonly recognised to be an important concept in understanding the experience of old age. This has been acknowledged in a number of studies. (For example, Lund, 1989; Essex and Klein, 1989). Major life changes such as bereavement, the onset of disability and institutionalisation have been shown to threaten a persons' sense of identity by destroying the basis on which their life is constructed. Taff (1985) in clarifying how ageing affects self-esteem draws on the concept of the 'looking glass self'. Perceptions of others act as mirrors reflecting images of self, this is the 'outer' self esteem and as such is based on approval and acceptance of others.

It's damned awful being a patient, you wish you were well. I don't think it's enjoyable but I mean a nurse can give a lot of comfort really.

The reader is likely to be very familiar with the influences on 'outer' self-esteem. Any older person today is aware of, and affected by, the overtly ageist society in which we live. In an attempt to counteract this ageism, nurses who work with older people must do so because they both like and value older people. It is not enough to call for positive attitudes, this implies that the nurse need do no more than apply 'politically' correct behaviour.

The impact of ageing on 'inner' self esteem relates to the amount of power and control older people are able to exert over their environment. It will have been influenced by their experiences throughout life. Some patients will have a high self-esteem and others will not.

Well you think, some of the young girls have got better ideas ... you know ... we've only got a few.

Those with a high self-esteem are likely to be clear about their role as a patient.

I'm not a perfect patient and I wouldn't want to be. But I think you've got your duty to people as they've got their duty to you. The nurses, who know a lot are very kind, but they don't know everything.

Confident people may well be confident patients. But the confidence is inevitably affected by the series of losses which normally precede entering a continuing care setting. Social exchange theory suggests that the relative power of older people is gradually diminished as a result of the decrease in social exchange relationships (Dowd, 1975). Whilst social exchange theory does not fully explain the impact of ageing it goes some way to offer insight into the importance of the nurse–resident relationship.

The nurse-resident relationship

Sociability

Good human relationships can be among our most valuable personal assets and gerontologists speculate that this is especially important to people in later life. Studies have focused on such relationships in terms of family (for example, Townsend, 1957); and family and friends (for example, Hawley and Chamley, 1986). For the participants of this study however, close relationships between patient and nurse clearly existed and were valued. General sociability was important, as cheerfulness and the use of humour.

Nurses' sociability makes a real difference to the quality of my life. Well to go about their job happy like ... you know whereas if they come along and they're grumpy and that sort of thing you think why are they like that to me?

In Donabedian's (1989) study, it was clear that the requirement for good relationships superseded the need for amenities and was more important than technical care though there was some suggestion that the latter was assumed to be always delivered. Recognition that nurses formed an important support system as part of the participants' social networks was evident.

Confidants

I don't want to be close with all the nurses, some are my friends and some are not.

A study by Huss (1988) explored patient satisfaction with nursing in American long-term facilities. Results indicated a significantly higher life satisfaction score for those patients who reported having a confidant. These findings are consistent with those reported by Lowenthal and Haven (1976). Nurses contribute to enhanced life satisfaction scores if their role is one of confidant. These studies suggest that the relationship between patient and nurse in continuing care settings may be very important. In the current study it is these relationships with nurses which the participants emphasise are of key importance.

Social networks

In an anthropological social network analysis, Powers (1992) studied the different ways health care residents (aged 55 years and over) interpret relationships with staff. The study identified that residents with low numbers of supportive networks on admission, turned to staff as a source of dependent support and emotional attachment. Whilst my study cannot draw comparisons, there is clear evidence from all four participants that they value close relationships with some of the nurses. Interestingly this did not appear to relate to the number of family and friends within the participants' social networks. It would seem that relationships may be the very essence of continuing care for older people.

Reciprocity

Therapeutic reciprocity describes an exchange between nurse and patient that is referenced both subjectively and objectively by personal and empirical data (Marck, 1990). By linking the concepts of partnership, intimacy and reciprocity, Meutzal (1988) demonstrates that it is valid for both the nurse and the patient to benefit from their relationship. Partnership is well established in British nursing literature as a desirable characteristic of the nurse–patient relationship. (For example, Pearson and Vaughan, 1986; Royal College of Nursing, 1987.) There is, however, no published evidence to suggest that older patients want to form partnerships with nurses. Nevertheless, King (1981) argues that reciprocity is an essential characteristic. The interactions between nurse and patient are fundamental; involving the patient and establishing a genuine relationship will enhance feelings of autonomy and security.

The social exchange theory of ageing described by Dowd (1975) examines causes and consequences of the disadvantaged power position of older people. If older people are no longer accorded the privilege of reciprocation and are left only with compliance and deference to bargain with, then loss of self-esteem will quickly follow.

The nurse symbolizes 'significant other' in the life of the patient:

> *She's like a mother to me.*

and,

> *I had ever such a long chat with her and I felt better. She understood me you know, really cares.*

This reliance on nurses in continuing care may result in the expectations of the nurse assuming great importance for the patient. Behaviour may accord with those expectations, especially if the patient feels so powerless that all they have to offer the relationship is compliance and good behaviour. The nurse must therefore facilitate reciprocity in the relationship. To be successful in such a reciprocal relationship the nurse contributes nursing knowledge, skills and self. The patient contributes personal knowledge about their needs and wants. It is the balance of the offering of self which changes the relationship from good to special.

I've got quite a few of the nurses to give up smoking.

The anthropological literature on ageing suggests that the need for reciprocation is universal for maintaining a strong sense of self-worth amongst older people (Jonas and Wellin, 1980). People helping people has been recognised as a valuable resource for all individuals. It is of particular significance for older members of society. For the nurse, knowledge is acquired by skilled efforts to understand from the client's perspective. At the expert level of practice this 'knowing' of a particular patient's perspective may be what the participants refer to as intuition. The knowledge received and acted upon by the nurse cannot necessarily be broken down and analysed.

Perhaps if nurses can truly acknowledge that the essence of health care is still something that happens between people, the power of caring can be extended through a recognition of the therapeutic and nurturing role of reciprocity. Nurses can affirm and assist clients' work, appreciate their agendas and establish the collaborative nurse–client relationship described in the literature. The nursing profession can risk the cost of caring to the mutual enrichment of patients and nurses.

Reflections on the findings

Older people who are patients in continuing care settings are some of the most highly dependent and disadvantaged members of society. This study demonstrates, however, that they have a clear view of what nurses and nursing means to them. They know what they want and what they value. Further studies would need to be conducted to ascertain whether these findings can be generalised. Mechanisms clearly need to be set up which will facilitate the gathering of such views. Such mechanisms would promote the concept of a consumer-led service.

The participants were able to distinguish between the different levels of knowledge and skills held by nurses. They showed clear insight in identifying the expert nurses. It is likely, therefore, that further studies on the value of nursing from the patient's perspective may shed useful insights and enhance the professional debates.

It has been suggested that continuing care patients do not require the services of qualified nurses. This study suggests otherwise. The participants gave clear accounts of why qualified nurses made a difference both in terms of technical care and their quality of life. Intuition exists, is recognised and is valued by the participants. The question, however, is can it be taught? To date there is no clear evidence either way but the literature suggests that the debate will continue in an effort to identify the attributes which will specify the value of nursing (for example Benner, 1984). The relationships between resident and nurse appear to have a greater influence on the resident's quality of life than any other factor. This suggests that greater emphasis on relationships should be incorporated in any quality audits being utilised and in educational programmes. It is clear that relationships are of key significance for the participant; this may be related to them being ongoing relationships. Perhaps patients could be involved in drawing up the criteria used to measure the quality of such services. It would be interesting to note the priority given to factors relating to relationships.

Caring is identified as an important component of the nurse–client relationship and there is an exhaustive professional literature on caring as a concept. In this study it is identified as expressions of love and affection. The caring gestures that make the participants feel qualitatively different are clearly described. Caring makes a difference and is valued, but it is still in danger of being marginalised.

The study has highlighted the acute feelings of vulnerability and powerlessness experienced. Such feelings are exacerbated by the series of losses which often precede admission to a continuing care ward. Nurses working in such settings will therefore need to be acutely aware of the effects of such losses. In highly dependent patients who have little control over their daily activities, being involved in making decisions about their care, the way the ward is decorated or what the new dog should be called, can therefore assume great importance. So will immediate attention in terms of meeting residents' needs. For example, for the patient who is totally reliant on nurses, prompt response to their requests for help will lessen the frustration of dependence. In contrast, the patient who is made to wait until the nurse is free is likely to express great frustration which the nurse may view as inappropriate behaviour. For the nurse who has been educated about the effects of dependency and powerlessness, who has undergone some experiential learning to help her understand, such expression of frustration will be more readily understood.

However, unless staffing levels reflect the needs of such dependent patients no amount of education will affect the quality of service provided. Building relationships calls for investment of time. The caring which has been identified as having such an impact on the participants' quality of life demands both personality attributes and the opportunity to express such caring. The 'attention to the little things' which was cited as being a clear indication of caring, takes time too. These are the things which all too often have to be sacrificed in the drive to provide a cost-effective service.

A particularly interesting finding is the participants' desire for a reciprocal relationship with the nurse. This is especially the case when nurses are identified as friends. Examples of what the participants offered the nurses range from: being a grateful and predictable patient, helping nurses to give up smoking, and sending a nurse some flowers. There are no clear indications that reciprocity is currently included in pre-registrations programmes nor in subsequent courses for qualified nurses. Indeed nurses are openly discouraged from accepting gifts. In the continuing care settings this is likely to marginalise the resident who may feel that they have little to offer the relationship unless gifts are accepted.

The study generates new knowledge in that it has asked patients what they value in nursing. It is suggested that patients in continuing care may particularly value relationships with nurses and that those relationships must be based on reciprocity. Such a small study can clearly not be generalised and recommendations for practice cannot be made. The study would need to be replicated. Such replication could lead to the development of a tool which may identify older residents' values in relation to nursing.

The value of this study is that individuals will interpret it, based on their own beliefs and values. It is not possible to recommend changes in nursing practice as a result of such a small study. There are, however, clear implications for patients, nurses, educators and managers. For example, if I was reading this as an older person, it might lead me to question how nurses are selected to work with older people. As a nurse it might help me understand why residents get so angry and frustrated when I cannot attend to their needs promptly. As a manager I might consider whether it is necessary to appoint staff who both like and have positive attitudes towards older people and whether there is a difference. As a nurse educator I might consider including the concept of reciprocity in the curriculum. Everyone therefore may draw different priorities and conclusions from this study; this is its potential strength. It is flexible enough for all interested parties to find meaning within it.

Reflections on the research method

In my attempts to ensure that the residents retained control over the research process, I made appointments verbally and confirmed arrangements with appointment cards. Having booked the sessions with them, the nurses, and in the diary, I sometimes arrived for the appointments to find that visitors had arrived unannounced. This reinforced with me how little control is offered to older people by visitors who assume that people are free all day because they live in a care environment. It struck me that this was an issue which needed to be addressed.

The research paticipants were involved in checking all the transcripts, and checking the findings at each stage of the complicated and rigourous steps of the analysis. It was important to involve them all the way through in order to ensure that the findings were always true to what they were saying, and never my own interpretation. Despite the research participants being some of the most highly dependent and disempowered members of society, the process proved to be an enriching and empowering experience for us all. The participants told me that they had enjoyed being involved, and saw their contribution as a way of helping older people. For me, involving the participants meant that I could fulfil my own personal nursing values of involving older people in my work.

Personal reflections

In addition to the challenges of the research method, undertaking the study was time-consuming and tiring. During the fieldwork I experienced role conflict. I was there as a researcher yet I am a nurse and have experience of counselling. I resisted the temptation to act out my role as a nurse. Ignoring my potential therapeutic role was more challenging. In one interview things were shared with me which the teller told for the first time; in two of the transcripts there were clear indications of unhappy life events. But they had nothing to do with the value of nursing and this particular study. A reflective diary and regular supervision helped alert me to this. Such reflections helped me accept that my study could only tell one story, that of what patients value in nursing.

Yet there is of course the story of individuality, the story of dependency, the story of reciprocity and the story of being a good patient. Perhaps the most powerful experience and lesson learnt was that I had not expected the role of researcher to feel so different from that of the nurse. As a researcher I had no right to be asking questions, no authority, no technical skill or previous knowledge. Perhaps this was a strength. It is possible that I related to the participants because of the vulnerability which I was experiencing. I was totally dependent on their good will. Just as they are totally dependent on the good will of nurses.

References

Altschul, A. (1972) Patient Nurse Interaction. University of Edinburgh, Department of Nursing Studies, Monograph No. 3, Edinburgh: Churchill Livingstone.

Anderson, B. (1987) What makes excellent nursing homes different from ordinary nursing homes? *Danish Medical Bulletin*, 5, 7 –11.

Audit Commission (1991) The Virtue of Patients: making the best use of ward nursing resources, London: HMSO.

Bagust, A. and Slack, R. (1991) *Ward Nursing Quality*: York Health Economics Consortium, University of York.

Bagust, A. Oakley, J. and Slack, R. (1992) Quality or Quantity, *Health Service Journal* 102 (August), 23–25.

Baker, D. (1983) 'Care' in the geriatric ward: an account of two styles of nursing. In J. Wilson-Barnett (ed.) *Nursing Research: ten studies in patient care*. Chichester: John Wiley.

Batchelor, I. (1984) Policies for Crisis? Some aspects of DHSS policies for care of the elderly, Occasional paper 1, Nuffield Provincial Hospitals Trust, Oxford.

Benner, P. (1984) *From Novice to Expert: Exellence and Power in Clinical Nursing Practice*. Menlo Park: Addison Wesley.

Benner, P. and Wrubel, J. (1989) Caring is the candle that lights the dark, that permits us to find answers where others see none, *American Journal of Nursing*, **8**, 1073–1075.

Bond, J. (1984) Evaluation of long stay accommodation for elderly people. In Bromley D. (ed.) *Gerontology: Social and Behavioural Perspectives*. London: Croom Helm.

Bond, J. and Bond, S. (1987) Developments in the provision and evaluation of long term care for dependent old people. In: P. Fielding, (ed.) *Research in nursing care of elderly people*. Chichester, John Wiley.

Bond, J., Bond, S., Donaldson, C. et al. (1989a) *Evaluation of an innovation in the continuing care of very frail elderly people*. Report No. 38, vol. 7. Health Care Research Unit, School of Health Care Studies, University of Newcastle upon Tyne.

Bond, J., Bond, S., Donaldson, C. et al. (1989b) Evaluation of an innovation in the continuing care of very frail elderly people. *Ageing and Society*, **9**, 347-381.

Bromley, D. (ed.) *Gerontology: social and behavioural perspectives*. London: Croom Helm.

Buchan, J. and Ball, J. (1991) *Caring costs: Nursing Costs and Benefits*. London Institute of Manpower studies.

Clark, P. and Bowling, A. (1989) Observational Study of Quality of Life in NHS Nursing Homes and a Long stay Ward for the Elderly. *Ageing and Society*, **9**(2), 123–148.

Cornwell, J. (1989) The Consumer's View: Elderly People and Community Health Services. London: King's Fund.

Cronin, S. and Harrison, B. (1988) The importance of nurse caring behaviours as percieved by patients after myocardial infarction. *Heart & Lung*, **17** (4), 374–380.

Department of Health (1989) Caring for People: community care in the next decade and beyond. London: HMSO.

Department of Health (1990) The NHS and Community Care Act. London: HMSO.

Department of Health (1991) The Patient's Charter. London: HMSO.

Donadedian, A. (1989) Institutional and professional responsibilities in Quality Assurance. *Quality Assurrance in Health Care*, **1**(1), 3–11.

Dowd, J. (1975) Ageing as exchange; a preface to theory. *Journal of Gerontology*, **30**, 584–594.

Ebrahim, S. (1993) Longterm Care for Elderly People. *Quality in Health Care*, **2**, 198–203.

Elander, G. (1993) Ethical dilemmas in long term care settings: interviews with nurses in Sweden and England. (Conflicts in caring for the elderly, and in the nurse patient relationship). *International Journal of Nursing* **30**(1), 91–97.

Essex, M. and Klein, M. (1989) The importance of self concept and coping responses in explaining physical health status and depression among older women, *Journal of Ageing and Health*, **1**, 327–348.

Graham, H.(1983) Caring: a labour of love: In J. Finch and D. Groves, (eds.) *A Labour of Love*. London: Routledge and Kegan Paul.

Hawley, P. and Chamley, J. (1986) Older Persons' Perceptions of the Quality of their Human Support Systems, *Ageing and Society*, **6**(3), 295–312.

Henwood, M. (1992) *Through a glass darkly: community care and elderly people*. London: Kings Fund Institute.

Huss, J., Buckwalter, K., Stolley, J. (1988) Nursing's impact on life satisfaction. *Journal of Gerontological Nursing*, **14**(5), 31–36.

Jonas, K. and Wellin, E. (1980) Dependency and reciprocity: Home health aid in an elderly population, In C. Fry, (ed.) *Aging in Culture and Society*. J.F. Bergin Publishers. New York: Brooklyn.

Jones, L., Leneman, L., Maclean, U. (1987) Consumer feedback for the N.H.S.: a litrerature review. London: King Edwards Hospital Fund.

King, I. (1981) *A Theory for Nursing Systems, Concepts, Process*. New York: John Wiley.

Larson, P.J. (1984) Important nurse caring behaviours perceived by patients with Cancer. *Oncology Nursing Forum*, **11**(6), 46–50.

Lund, D. (ed.) (1989) Older Bereaved Spouses: Research with Practical Applications. New York: Hemisphere.

Loveredge, C. and Heineken, J. (1988) Confirming interactions, (Nurse patient relationships) *Journal of Gerontological Nursing*, **14**(5) May 23–26.

Lowenthal, M. and Haven, C. Interaction and adaption, intimacy as critical variable, (1976) In. R. Atchley, and M. Seltzer, (eds.) *Sociology of Aging: selected readings*. Belmont, California: Woodsworth Publishing. pp. 45–52.

Mangold, A. (1991) Senior nursing students' and professional nurses' perceptions of effective caring behaviours, a comparative study, *Journal of Nurse Education*, **30**(3), 134–139.

Marck, P. (1990) Therapeutic Reciprocity: a caring phenomenon. *Advanced Nursing Science*, **13**(1), 49–59.

Meutzal, P. (1988) Therapeutic nursing. In A. Pearson (ed.) *Primary Nursing: Nursing in the Burford and Oxford Nursing Development units*. London: Croom Helm.

Oliver, S. and Redfern, S. (1992) Interpersonal communication between nurses and elderly patients: refinement of an observation schedule, (research). *Journal of Advanced Nursing*, **16**(1) Jan. 30–38.

Paterson, J. and Zderad, L. (1976) *Humanistic Nursing*, New York: John Wiley and Sons.

Peace, S., Hall, J.F., Hamblin, G. (1979) The Quality of life of the elderly in residential care: a feasibility study, Research report No. 1, Survey Research Unit, Polytechnic of North London.

Peace, S. (1993) Quality of Institutional Life. Reviews in *Clinical Gerontology*, **3**(2), 187–193.

Pearson, A. and Vaughan, B. (1986) *Nursing Models for Practice*. London: Heinemann.

Pembry, S. (1984) Nursing Care: professional progress. *Journal of Advanced Nursing*, **9**(6) 539–547.

Powers, B. (1992) The roles staff play in the social networks of elderly institutionalized people. *Social Science and Medicine*, **34**(12) 1335–1343.

Raphael, W. (1965) Patient Care, Patients and staff; their likes and dislikes. *Nursing Times*, **61**, 1654–1656.

Rew, L. and Barton, M. (1989) Nurses' Intuition, *AORN Journal*, **50**, 353–358.

Risser, N. (1975) Development of an instrument to measure patient satisfaction with nurses and nursing care in primary care settings. *Nursing Research*, **24**(1), 45–52.

Rosenthal, K. (1992) Coronary Care Patients' and Nurses' perceptions of important nurse caring behaviors, *Heart and Lung, Journal of Critical Care*, Nov./Dec. **21**(6) 536–539.

Royal College of Nursing (1987) *Improving the care of elderly people in hospital*. Joint working party: British Geriatric Society, Royal College of Psychiatrists and Royal College of Nursing. London: RCN.

Royal College of Nursing (1992) *The Value of Nursing*, London: RCN.

Royal College of Nursing (1993a) Older People and Continuing Care. *The skill and value of the nurse*, Oct. London: RCN.

Royal College of Nursing (1993b) *The Value and Skill of Nurses working with Older People*, Nov. London: RCN.

Sinclair, I. (1988) Residential care for elderly people. In I. Sinclair (ed.) *Residential Care: the research reviewed* (The Wagner Report) London: HMSO.

Sixsmith, A. (1986) Independence and home in later life. In C. Phillipson, M. Bernard and P. Strang, (eds.) *Dependency and Interdependency in Old Age; theoretical perspectives and policy alternatives*. Beckenham: Croom Helm.

Smith, P. (1992) *The emotional Labour of Nursing*. Basingstoke: Macmillan.

Taff, L. (1985) Self Esteem in Later Life: a nursing perspective. *Advanced Nursing Science*, **8**(1) 77–84.

Thorne, S. and Robinson, C. (1988) Legacy of the country doctor. *Journal of Gerontological Nursing*, **14**(5) 23–26.

Thorne, S. and Robinson, C. (1989) Guarded Alliance: Health Care Relationships in Chronic Illness. *Image: Journal of Nursing Scholarship*, **21**(3) 153–157.

Townsend, P. (1957) *The Family Life of Old People*. London: Routledge and Kegan Paul.

Ungerson, C. (1983a) Why do women care? In J. Finch and D. Groves (eds.) *A Labour of Love*. London: Routledge and Kegan Paul.

Ungerson, C. (1983b) Women and caring: skills, tasks and taboos. In E. Gamarnikov, Morgan, D., Purvis, J. et al. (eds.) *The Public and The Private*. London: Heinemann, pp. 62–77.

Ungerson, C. (1990) The Language of Care. In C. Ungerson (ed.) *Gender and Caring*. London: Harvester/Wheatsheaf.

University of York Centre (1992) Skill Mix and the effectiveness of nursing care. University of York.

Von Essen, L. and Sjoden (1991) The importance of nurse care behaviours as perceived by Swedish hospital patients and nursing staff. *International Journal of Nursing Studies*, **28**(3), 267–281.

Wade, B., Sawyer, L., Bell, J. (1983) Dependency with dignity. Occasional Papers in social administration, No. 68. London: Bedford Square Press.

Wenger, C. (1989) Support Networks in Old Age: Constructing a typology. In M. Jeffrey, (ed.) *Growing old in the Twentieth Century.* London: Routledge.

Willcocks, D., Peace, S. Kellaher, L. et al. (1982) The residential life of old people: a study in 100 Local Authority Homes, 1. Polytechnic of North London, Survey Research Unit, Research Report No. 12.

Quality of Life Matters

5

Life Transitions

Brendan McCormack

> All our lives long, every day and every hour, we are engaged in the process of accommodating our changed and unchanged selves to changed and unchanged surroundings; living, in fact is nothing else than this process of accommodation. When we fail in it a little we are stupid, when we fail flagrantly we are mad, when we suspend it temporarily we sleep, when we give up the attempt altogether, we die.
>
> (from Samuel Butler, cited in Golan, 1981)

This chapter will explore the psychological, physical and social effects of ageing through developing our understanding of the meanings of age and ageing to older people. The chapter develops the idea of the older person moving through a journey of dependence while seeking his or her own identity, individuality and independence. It will explore the idea of the ageing body in transition, seeking a place of healing where the many roles of life can be played out to the end. It will consider the role of the nurse as an enabler, working alongside the older person. The chapter proposes that nursing in care home settings should endeavour to restore the pride and self-esteem that may have been eroded as a result of illness, disability or ageing.

> Growing old well is about letting go of youth and accepting whatever comes next. The nature of life is change. The nature of growth is change.
>
> (Taylor, 1992)

The Community Care Act is now well established, with its central aim of encouraging vulnerable people to live as independently as possible in their own homes if they choose to do so. For those who cannot, then care homes will be an option. The current and projected rise in the numbers of those aged 75 years and over will continue to be a cause for celebration as well as a challenge for resource allocations in both health and social services. Inevitably this will impact upon the care home sector, although some provision of continuing care in a home is always likely to be needed. It can also be assumed that the majority (if not all) of continuing care will be provided in care home settings as we continue to see the reduction of NHS-funded continuing care facilities alongside over-stretched community services.

The meaning of old age

> Being old is not some kind of illness but a position of pride and respect that you have earned. People should want to be old. They should look forward to it.
>
> (Taylor, 1992)

What to do we mean when we ask how old a person is? What is behind the question that we are asking? Do we wish to know about the person's chronological age, psychological age, emotional age or social age? Or are we simply reinforcing stereotypes about what is acceptable behaviour at a particular age? Age does correlate with many of the changes that occur through natural ageing, and therefore is important to consider when making care decisions. However, it is these 'ageing factors' that should be considered in care decisions and not chronological age alone. There are many theories for ageing (see for example Hendricks and Hendricks, 1977), but what is common among all of them is that the concept of age is difficult to define because it has many differing meanings. Physiologically, different parts of the body age at different rates, as do an individual's ability to deal with things and cope with social change. Thus, it is possible to be 'old' according to the calendar, yet have the heart of a middle aged adult and the emotions of a teenager. Interpretations of one's age are always subjective, and may be influenced by other factors such as family life, career or health status.

Deteriorating physical circumstances offer a daily reminder of the body's limitations to the outside world. Feelings of alienation can result in individuals seeing themselves as less of a person and more like an object. Such feelings can limit the person's connection with the outside world. This may be exaggerated by the media's worship of youth and beauty, obsession with a fast-paced lifestyle and emphasis on efficiency and productivity. Instead of viewing old age as a valuable, final culmination of the life span, society promotes a stereotyped view of ageing as less than normal.

The denial of sexuality in older people is one common example. Some of us hope that sex won't rear its ugly head in patients and residents, and even if it does we would rather translate the sexual needs of older people as social needs because it's more comfortable for us. A recent story of a family trying to find a suitable nursing home placement for their parents epitomised this attitude. The couple had never slept apart from each other except for periods of hospitalisation and therefore wanted a room together with a double bed facility. The difficulties experienced by the family in finding such a place were enormous, as the logic consisted of: if the couple were well enough to sleep together, then did they really need care in a nursing home?!

The concept of transitions

The word 'transition' is defined as a 'passage from one place, state, stage, style or subject to another' (Chambers, 1989). Because such definitions include aspects of both time and movement, a transition can be thought of as a process of psychological adaptation whereby a change in circumstances is linked to experienced movement. For example, the older person deciding to move to a nursing home is experiencing a change in circumstance (the decision to give up one's own home) and move to a new state of dependence.

Transitions can then be seen as passages from one life phase, condition, or status to another, incorporating elements of process (how the transition is managed), time span (the time it takes to move to a new state) and perception (our beliefs and values about the transition and our desire for it to occur) (Chick and Meleis, 1986). Therefore a transition will occur if a change or disruption to a person's reality necessitates a reorganisation of that reality (Selder, 1989), as illustrated in Figure 5.1.

Reality refers to our everyday world. Each individual's reality has values which are essential to the way the person sees themselves and their world. Many aspects of an individual's reality may be shared with others, so that common understandings can exist in a sense of community. However, it is the individuality of our personal meanings that determines 'who I am'. As life progresses we establish our personal identity, creating the foundations on which the stable structures of one's life are built. If these structures are challenged in any way, through bereavement for example, then the once stable foundation becomes unstable and the structures of one's life may fall or crumble. The disruption that occurs will continue until stability in the new circumstances is achieved.

Some transitions may be planned, such as retirement. Other transitions occur suddenly and without opportunity to make preparations, such as an acute health crisis. However, in both cases a transition is initiated because the person's current reality (circumstance) is disrupted. Individuals differ in their ability to adapt to such disruption. In many cases the transition to nursing home care will occur with ease as the older person recognises the need for care and support and identifies the potential for new opportunities, while for others it may signify failure, despair and loss of identity. However the individual copes with their change of reality, the transition requires the person to adapt and this will occur over a period of time. The 'stages of death' model offered by Kubler-Ross (1969) describes a process of adaptation that may be experienced by people who are dying. She identifies five stages of adaptation:

1. denial and isolation;
2. anger and resentment;
3. bargaining;
4. depression, and
5. acceptance.

It has been suggested that the individual moves through the five stages in a dynamic way. Such a model should, however, only be used as a guide. Not everyone will go through these stages and certainly will not necessarily go through them in the order that Kubler-Ross (1969)

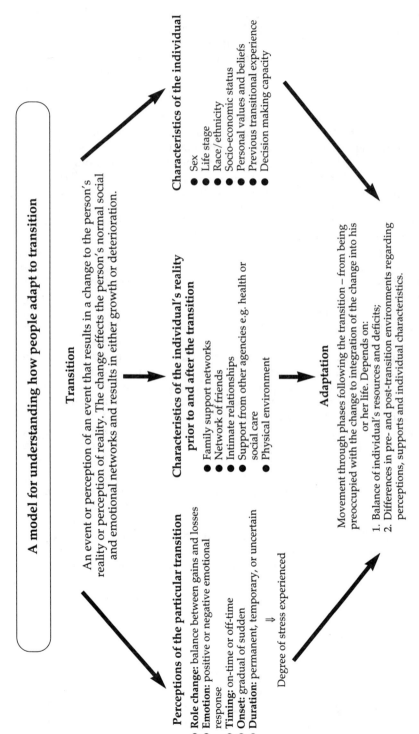

A model for understanding how people adapt to transition

Transition

An event or perception of an event that results in a change to the person's reality or perception of reality. The change effects the person's normal social and emotional networks and results in either growth or deterioration.

Characteristics of the individual

- Sex
- Life stage
- Race/ethnicity
- Socio-economic status
- Personal values and beliefs
- Previous transitional experience
- Decision making capacity

Characteristics of the individual's reality prior to and after the transition

- Family support networks
- Network of friends
- Intimate relationships
- Support from other agencies e.g. health or social care
- Physical environment

Perceptions of the particular transition

- **Role change:** balance between gains and losses
- **Emotion:** positive or negative emotional response
- **Timing:** on-time or off-time
- **Onset:** gradual or sudden
- **Duration:** permanent, temporary, or uncertain
  ⇒
  Degree of stress experienced

Adaptation

Movement through phases following the transition – from being preoccupied with the change to integration of the change into his or her life. Depends on:

1. Balance of individual's resources and deficits;
2. Differences in pre- and post-transition environments regarding perceptions, supports and individual characteristics.

Figure 5.1   *(adapted from Schlossberg, 1981)*

suggests. As the older person adapts to living in a care home, not only does the individual experience considerable change, but the lives of family members, significant others and carers are affected. The extent of the change experienced depends on the roles and relationships in place prior to the transition:

> At the onset of chronic illness, the individual must focus attention on the process of acquiring new roles or role modifications, interpersonal interactions, and associations, the development of new self definitions, the learning of new skills, and suitable self-fulfilling and satisfying activities all part of grief resolution.
>
> (Werner-Beland, 1980)

However, even if we accept the notion that adaptation to transition may follow a particular pattern, the question of why some people adapt more quickly and easily than others remains unanswered. It may be that the conditions before and after the transition and the person's sense of competence, well-being and health are key indicators of adaption.

For example:

> Joan and Brigid are two patients on a rehabilitation ward being faced with the reality that they will require long term care in the future. They are both trying to come to terms with their disabilities following a stroke. For both of them it is a psychologically and socially painful prospect. Joan however has ample resources to balance the deficit – she is a determined woman who has always been in control of her own affairs. She has a supportive family who are committed to finding Joan the home that exactly suits her values and needs. She also has the financial security to make such decisions. She further believes that life will be easier for her in a care home as she won't have to worry about the 'daily drudges' of life but instead can concentrate on her own particular interests. She has for some time found maintaining her large Victorian property to be too much for her.
>
> Brigid however has low resources at this time in her life. She finds the daily help she needs intolerable as she has always been a private person. Her husband had previously been the only person to see her naked and she now feels 'dirty' and 'undignified' because of her circumstances. However, her husband is dead and her speech problems prevent her from being able to explain to the nurses her beliefs and values. She is financially insecure and will have to rely on the State to pay for her care. She has heard 'bad reports' about the home she is being moved to, but because of a lack of available places elsewhere she knows she has to accept it. Therefore, the deficits far outweigh the resources in Brigid's case.

What these examples demonstrate is the importance of addressing the issue of resources and deficits when considering how well a person will adapt to change. It further begins to clarify why two people may adapt to the same transition in very different ways. Such considerations are essential when assisting the older person make the transition from independent living to continuing care.

The body in transition

The older person is moving through a journey of dependence while seeking their own identity and individuality. This sense of 'seeking the individual', brings their past to the older person, in order to create a future. The care home is a new experience, assimilated by the influence of their past and their aspirations for the future. As we move through the life-span, we experience many different goals, ambitions and desires.

The romance of youth often changes to the chaos of adulthood and finally to a time when we wish to seek out the meaning of our lives. It is sadly true that at the time when life can have the most meaning, it is often the time that has greatest loss:

> One day you're an attractive alluring woman and the next day you become one of the faceless group of old ladies who sit alone in cafes and on park benches. One of the wrinklies, shrinklies, crumblies, old bags, old bats – bewildered at the speed of the descent, dismissed as irrelevant, dying of loneliness. With no recognised rites of passage, we grope uneasily in the frightened tunnel of transition, unsure of what lies ahead, afraid to relinquish what has gone before.
>
> (Taylor, 1992)

Transition of home

The loss of individuality through disability and illness which is often experienced through the ultimate sacrifice of losing one's home, can lead to a loss of identity. The depersonalisation of the individual that occurs in institutional settings is well documented (e.g.: Goffman, 1961; Miller and Gwynne, 1972; Kenny, 1990). The central feature of this institutionalisation is the creation of dependence. Goffman's work eloquently describes how this process occurs, with the chief cause being the breakdown of the barriers normally separating the three spheres of life, i.e. sleep, play and work. Instead, all aspects of life are conducted in the same surroundings, in the public eye of the same authority, with others who are pursuing the same thing at the same time. The activities of the day are tightly scheduled within an explicit set of rules and boundaries.

Having entered the institution with certain self-conceptions made possible by certain social arrangements in the social world of his or her home (Kenny, 1990), the person is stripped of the support provided by such arrangements. Or as Goffman (1961) asserts 'he or she begins a series of abasements, degradations, humiliations and profanations of self'. When care home residents realise that they are no longer part of their human world, they experience despair (Royal College of Nursing, 1993). These feelings of such despair may be manifested through non-specific complaints of physical or psychological distress and the resident may be stereotyped as hypochondriacal, mentally unstable, depressed or just a 'complainer' (Royal College of Nursing, 1993). Kastenbaum (1983) demonstrated how these residents may subsequently be ignored by staff, neglected, ridiculed or given drugs – the symptoms are treated rather than the emotional distress. Dependence on others creates a form of learned helplessness.

It is not uncommon for young or middle-aged people to feel a sense of superiority over the old and frail. The slowness of movement, the hanging on to the past, old fashioned habits and the perceived unacceptance with the present world often contribute to this sense of superiority. So even if we aim to prevent institutionalisation occurring we can still feel a sense of sentimental pity towards the old when they are unable to share the haste and superficiality of our daily lives (Moody, 1991), again promoting a form of learned helplessness.

The meaning of life for older people is not demonstrated through the tedium of superficial daily life. Current approaches to reminiscence and life review attempts to aid an understanding of the meaning of life through a wish to find in the experience of older people, elements of strength and positive affirmation. Even though life around the person may have little meaning or significance, through individual life review, the person may discover meaning in their own life. Assisting the individual to find this meaning, may help them to tolerate the incongruity of their current situation and help create a future. As Moody (1991) asserts, 'if my life is intelligible, my life has purpose and my hopes and desires ultimately can be satisfied, then happiness can be found';

> At first we want life to be romantic; later, to be bearable; finally, to be understandable.
>
> (Bogan, cited in Moody, 1991)

Easing the transition

The consideration of a care home placement can be very emotionally charged and complex. Placing a loved one in a home can evoke familial guilt, anger and resentment and the family member being placed may also feel helpless, abandoned and rejected (Brody, 1977). The situation is not helped by the negative image of care homes that still prevails in our society, the financial reality of the decision with the ensuing loss of the home identity, and the reality that the conditions in some care homes are far from desirable. Good care home placement requires acknowledgement of the problems and difficulties such a decision entails. Older people and their families deserve to have the best possible professional interventions as they struggle to make decisions about placing their loved ones in care homes. Further, there is a need to understand the physical alteration that accompanies growing old and the problems that this poses. The loss that is threatened with ageing is not the sheer fact of physical decline, but the inevitable alienation from a body that is regarded as an imprisoning object (Gadow, 1991).

So, what implications does this have for nursing practice in the nursing home? The approach to care offered here is based on the humanistic principles of preserving the integrity of the person and the promotion of independence as illustrated in Figure 5.2 (adapted from O'Berle and Davies, 1992; Hutchinson and Bahr, 1991).

Healing environment

Central to this approach is the aim of providing a healing environment. Such a healing environment is not achieved by the emphasis on 'hygienic factors' alone (Miller and Gwynne, 1972). While the provision of comfortable, pleasant and homely living conditions goes some way towards the creation of a healing environment, the relationship between patient and carer can guarantee it. However this is not a one-way relationship, i.e. nurse to patient, but is indeed a reciprocal relationship where both parties grow as a result of the relationship.

Growth through learning, challenge and the expression of emotions aids the development of qualities of imagination, compassion and self-realisation in practice. This relationship establishes a personal–professional connection based on mutual respect and honesty (Genevay and Katz, 1990). Therefore humanistic nursing is itself a kind of healing art, a clinical art that is creative. It involves 'being with' and 'doing with', through the active participation of the patient in order to activate the potential within themselves.

The concept of 'total environment' that the care setting can offer, is central to this healing community. The older person's surroundings and approaches to their care should recognise their unique journey, which began with their detachment from their home environment. To an older person, their own home and the presence of a clutter of familiar possessions helps to preserve a sense of security and orientation in a world that moves too fast. It may be that older people are disturbed by changes in their physical environment as much as they are about loss of contact with friends or family. The environment of the nursing home should avoid making premature assumptions about people. Their new 'home' should offer a stability in which the person can find their unique individuality within it. An objective understanding of the ageing body, an understanding of the individual's subjective interpretation of their own ageing journey and the individual meanings attached contributes to a sense of wholeness and allows the nurse to enter the subjective world of the older person to meet care needs. Acceptance of the older person's life ways is

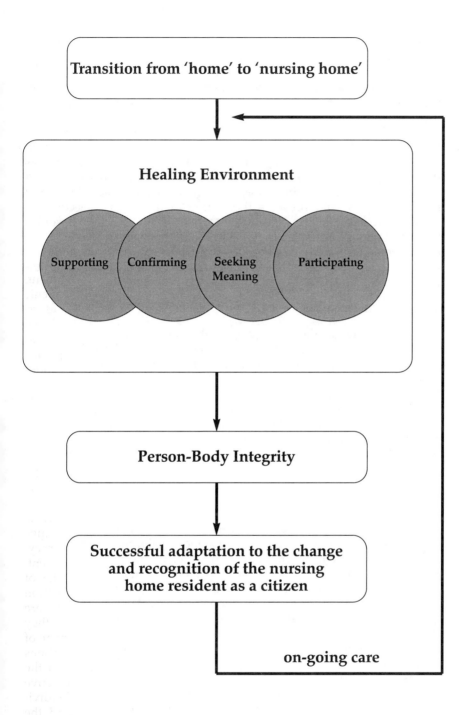

Figure 5.2   *Easing the transition (adapted from O'Berle and Davies, 1992 and Hutchinson and Bahr, 1991)*

perhaps one of the most humanistic qualities shown in nursing care. The older person is mindful of the many roles played during life and the losses suffered over the years.

To have a nurse show, through acceptance of the person, an empathic understanding of the patient's losses and present limitations, is to establish a therapeutic relationship which is directed at gaining an effective outcome from care that is centred on the person's needs and life perspectives. This understanding of the person's self-worth directs the nurse towards a flexibility in nursing care that seeks to preserve the integrity of the person. It also, through the appreciation of the individual's uniqueness, makes explicit to the nurse, the limits beyond which the person cannot be taken and prevents the setting of unrealistic objectives. If nursing older people is to be directed towards a humanistic philosophy, then as many opportunities as possible should be made available for the older person to exercise freedom of choice, take risks, express opinions, make decisions and be listened to! The according of such respect to the older person can in itself offer an approach to the 'healing' of the body and the restoration of individual self-worth. As another of Taylor's acquaintances proclaimed:

> As older women we are a considerable force once we own our strength. We can use it by becoming teachers. Acknowledge that you have a sense of destiny, that you know who you are and have something to say, Say it! You may be a film-maker or a writer. You may want to stand on a box and shout about it, you may make a basket or weave a rug. At whatever level, be a teacher – an exemplar. Say I have done something worthwhile with my life and I count.
>
> (Taylor, 1992)

Supporting

To be supportive, the nurse must believe in the inherent worth of the recipients of care and in their strengths and capabilities. Central to this notion of support is the fundamental belief in the autonomy of the patient. In a continuing care context, promoting individual autonomy is a dynamic and interrelated partnership between nurse and resident. It should not be based on assumptions about what the person might want to do, nor on the desire to protect the rights of individuals to 'do what they want'. But it is the effort to help persons become clear about what they want to do, by helping them discern their values in the situation.

It is only through the confirmation of their values that a person's decision can be self-determined. Once the decision has been made, it is therefore the role of the nurse to provide the support necessary for the person to reach the desired goal(s). This calls for expertise in flexibility and creativity in nursing care. The nurse facilitates coping and reinforces normality in daily life. Such activities as providing comfort measures and preserving the person's integrity during periods of pain and distress; providing appropriate, accurate and timely information; providing emotional support during developmental changes; and presencing – the art of 'being with' a person without the need to be 'doing to' the person (Benner, 1984), are all essential features of the nurse's supportive role. Further, the nurse needs skills in:

- assessing the older person's competence to make decisions;
- assessing the degree of risk involved in exercising such decision-making capacity;
- respecting the individual's right to make decisions;
- honouring such decisions once they have been made.

A nurse who thus allows herself to respond to the individuality of each person, will in some way allow herself to be a different nurse to each person. She will also find herself changing with time as expertise in facilitating decision-making grows and develops and in response to the changing needs of individuals.

Confirming

One of the most effective ways nurses can demonstrate caring to others, is through behaviours that express a way of confirming another as a respected and cared about human being. Respecting self-worth flows from the realisation of the many years of experience that may be lying dormant in the older person.

Restoration of self-worth through the experience of respect from others can bring about a form of healing in itself. Confirming, also includes recognising the health potential of the person irrespective of their current health state.

Health seen as 'potential' (Seedhouse, 1986) prevents fatalism in approaches to care, demonstrated through negative nursing behaviours of apathy and neglect, with the underlying assumption being that as older people are unwilling/unable to change old behaviours or learn new ones, health promotion is not relevant (Royal College of Nursing, 1993). However, it has been demonstrated that health promotion activities with older people can be effective in maximising wellness and reducing risk factors, through such activities as physical exercise and dietary regimes (Gray, 1982; Kane and Kane, 1983).

During the process of confirming, those who care and those who are cared for don't have to relate to each other as strong and weak, but both can grow in each other's capacity to learn from each other as equals. Therefore the focus is on helping the older person to look at him/herself in the context of a citizen of the home, rather than through the limited context of a patient. Specific activities that enable such a philosophy include:

- collaborative care planning between nurse and resident;
- Residents' committees;
- individual and group exercise programmes;
- movement to music;
- reminiscence activities, and
- story telling and life history groups.

Seeking meaning

Seeking meaning involves helping the person make sense out of what is happening to them in their world. The emphasis is on helping the person cope with the loss of his or her social identity and make the transition to their new world. It avoids making assumptions about the individual or the imposition of rules and regulations before the individual has established their own identity. The nurse, in being with the person, seeks to determine the personal meaning which the experience of illness, suffering or dying is to have for that individual (Gadow, 1980). Ultimately, the individual's self-determination means understanding the meaning of an experience, before decisions are reached about how best to respond practically to the experience.

The importance of approaching assessment from the patient's perspective is paramount. If the focus of assessment of older people's needs is based purely on the functional assessment of activities of daily living, then an understanding of the person's uniqueness can never be gained. Is that person really just a collection of body systems that all meet together conveniently, and, on the basis that one or more of them has malfunctioned, thus requires care? ... or alternatively is that person a unique individual who has marked out a unique journey in order to reach this stage of their life and now requires help to move on to the next stage?

By taking a biographical approach to assessment the nurse can establish a 'picture' that is individual and unique. A person's biography can be seen as an account of a number of separate but related life events that have influenced and directed the person's life. It is the history which gives meaning to the values of the individual and provides the explanations which are needed when crises occur and care decisions are being chosen (Johnson, 1991).

Indeed Schofield (1994) suggests that an experienced nurse will be able to recognise when biographical details are important to clarify concerns in care, thereby identifying the appropriate focus of care and the maintenance of the person's integrity.

Participating

It could be asserted that 'doing for' people is what we do best! However, the negative connotations that are associated with such activity usually equate with paternalistic nursing practice, whereby the older person is passive and the nurse is active. It often implies that the 'nurse knows best', is in the best position to make decisions for the resident and can therefore perform the activity on behalf of that person. We would surely all agree that in continuing care, there is a preponderance of physical care activities because of the client population and focus. However, this does not imply passivity on the part of the resident.

Wade (1983) describes an approach to care in long-term facilities that is characterised by consultation and involvement of the residents in their care programme. Their adulthood is recognised and every effort is made to maximise their physical and mental independence. This active involvement provides a form of rehabilitation that is aimed at improving functional independence, improving competence in self-care activities, preventing secondary complications, and promoting psychological well-being, confidence and self-esteem (Royal College of Nursing, 1993). In our current finance-driven world, savings in care staff time, pressure area treatments, wound dressings, incontinence pads, mobility aids and drugs could also be made through an emphasis on rehabilitation. Admission and continuing assessments of people's needs should include an evaluation of how the person could or does function in a socially productive manner, in addition to the typical focus on problems, pathology and losses (Hutchinson and Bahr, 1991).

Person–body integrity

As has already been discussed, the experience of disability can create a dissonance between the person and the body. The nurse is in the unique position of bridging these extremes and creating harmony and integrity. The nurse can assist the individual to understand their body, accept it as their own and 'live it' instead of allowing it to remain alien. The nurse becomes a professional friend and the nurse–resident relationship assumes some of the qualities usually described as part of a socially meaningful relationship. Many usual nursing tasks remain important, as it is through these that the physical needs of the person are met. But, as a friend, the nurse needs to know herself, what she is able to give and when to draw the line. Acceptance of individuality and being reflective about practice are fundamental to developing flexible approaches to care decisions. At its simplest level, the nurse needs to ask herself two fundamental questions:

1. Is the resident's individuality being respected and preserved, or overlooked and intruded upon?
2. Who is dictating the direction of the decision-making process at this moment, and why?

When a nurse goes more by the older person's direction and less by her own particular agenda or that of the organisation, it becomes easier to notice when the person is feeling out of tune with what is being planned and the direction that he/she is being taken. Unquestioning acceptance of organisational constraints on individuality is no excuse for the erosion of the person's ability to exercise their full decision-making potential.

Working with an older person in this way can be thought of as a mutual process of learning, or as Casement (1988) sees it, 'I as a nurse am learning from the patient'. If a nurse can trust in the relationship she has with a patient, then it is good to be led by the patient, not in a passive sense of 'being led' but in a dynamic sense where the cues and nuances of the patient's behaviour direct the focus of the action that needs to be taken. The patient is thus given a real part to play in helping the nurse discover new ways of working and a real partnership is established. Fresh insights emerge and the tendency to fall back onto old ritualised practices is avoided. There are of course other times when a firmness in approach has to be taken and sometimes without this firmness the person would feel insecure and at risk. However, as long as the reasons for this are made clear in the plan of care, partnership can still be maintained. The supporting, confirming, participating and seeking approaches to care create this person–body integrity.

Conclusion

What is being suggested here is that the total person needs to be understood when nurses and others work with older people. We need to adopt approaches to nursing that focus on people and their life ways. As nurses we need to be able to learn from older people in order to create the appropriate care environment. Older people should not 'suffer' because of the care they receive from nurses. Humanistic nursing tries to give the older person as many opportunities as possible to exercise freedom of choice, to express opinions, to make decisions, to talk while the nurse really listens and to have the opportunity to express their authentic self. To this end I could do no better than quote the words of Isaiah Berlin (1969) and hope and trust that this philosophy holds central to all our practice:

> I wish to be an instrument of my own, not other men's acts of will. I wish to be a subject, not an object … deciding, not being decided for, self directed and not acted upon by external nature or by other men as if I were a thing, or an animal, or a slave incapable of playing a human role, that is, conceiving goals and policies of my own and realising them … I wish to be somebody, not nobody.
>
> (Isaiah Berlin, 1969)

References

Benner, P. (1984) *From Novice to Expert: Excellence and Power in Clinical Nursing Practice*. Addison–Wesley.

Berlin, I. (1969) *Four Essays on Liberty*. Oxford University Press.

Brody, E. (1977) *Long term care of older people: A practical guide*. Human Services Press.

Casement, P. (1988) *On Learning from the Patient*. Tavistock Publications.

Chambers English Dictionary. Chambers (1989).

Chick, N. and Meleis, A.I. (1986) Transitions: A Nursing Concern. In P.L. Chinn (ed.) *Nursing Research Methodology – Issues and Implementation*. Aspen Publishers.

Gadow, S. (1980) Existential Advocacy: Philosophical Foundations of Nursing. In S.F. Spicker and S. Gadow (eds) *Nursing: Images and Ideals: Opening Dialogue with the Humanities*. Springer.

Genevay, B. and Katz, R.S. (1990) *Countertransference and Older Clients*. Sage.

Goffman, E. (1961) *On the Characteristics of Total Institutions. First Essay in Asylums*. Penguin.

Golan, N. (1981) *Passing Through Transitions – a guide for practitioners*. Collier Macmillan Publishers.

Gray, J.A. (1982) Practising prevention in old age. *British Medical Journal*, **285**, 545–547.

Hendricks, J. and Hendricks, C.D. (1977) *Ageing in Mass Society – myths and realities*. Winthrop Publishers.

Hunter, D.J. (1992) The prospects for long-term care: current policy and realistic alternatives. In L. Gormally (ed.) *The Dependent Elderly: Autonomy, Justice and Quality of Care*. Cambridge University Press.

Hutchinson, C.P. and Bahr, R.T. (1991) Types and Meanings of Caring Behaviours Among Elderly Nursing Home Residents. *IMAGE*, **23**, No. 2, 85–88.

Johnson, M.L. (1991) The meaning of old age. In S.J. Redfern (ed.) *Nursing Elderly People*. Churchill Livingstone.

Kane, R.L. and Kane, R.A. (1983) Predicting the outcomes in nursing home patients. *Gerontologist*, **23**, No. 2, 200-206.

Kastenbaum, R. (1983) Can the clinical milieu be therapeutic? In G.D. Rowles and A.R.J. Ohta (eds) *Ageing and Milieu: Environmental Perspectives on Growing Old*. Academic Press.

Kenny, T. (1990) Erosion of Individuality in care of elderly people in hospital – an alternative approach. *Journal of Advanced Nursing*, **15**, 571–576.

Kubler-Ross, E. (1969) *On Death and Dying*. Macmillan.

Miller, E. and Gwynne, G.A. (1972) *Life Apart*. A Pilot Study of Residential Institutions for the Physically Handicapped and Young Sick. Tavistock.

Moody, H.R. (1991) The Meaning of Life in Old Age. In N.S. Jecker (ed.) *Ageing and Ethics*. Humana Press.

O'Berle, K. and Davies, B. (1992) Supporting and Caring: Exploring the Concepts. *Oncology Nursing Forum*. **19**, No. 5, 763–767.

Royal College of Nursing (1993) *Older People and Continuing Care – The Skill and value of the Nurse*. RCN.

Sacks, O. (1991) *A Leg to Stand On*. Pan Books.

Schlossberg, N.K. (1981) A model for analyzing human adaptation to transition. *The Counselling Psychologist*, **9**(2), 2–18.

Schofield, I. (1994) An historical approach to care. *Elderly Care*, **6**, No. 6, 14–15.

Seedhouse, D. (1986) *Health: the foundations of achievement*. John Wiley and Sons.

Selder, F. (1989) Life Transition Theory: the resolution of uncertainty, *Nursing and Health Care*, **10**, No. 8, 437–451.

Taylor, A. (1992) *Older Than Time*. Harper Collins Publishers.

Wade, B. (1983) Different models of care for the elderly. *Nursing Times*, **79**, No. 12.

Werner-Beland, J.A. (ed.) (1980) *Grief responses to long-term illness and disability*. Reston Publishing Company.

World Health Organisation (1989) *Health of the Elderly*. Technical Report Series 779, WHO.

6

Rights, Risks and Responsibilities

Hazel Heath

Introduction

It could be argued that all citizens, regardless of their age and health status, should have the same rights, duties and responsibilities as others. Yet in the day to day reality of care homes, even the nurses who are wholeheartedly committed to these values and principles can find that putting them into practice is less than straightforward. The rights of older people who are physically frail can easily become eroded if others carry out their activities of living for them. Older people who are mentally frail are even more at risk of losing their rights, as assumptions are made about what they would want, or what is best for them. Nurses and other professionals may make decisions with the best of intentions, such as to protect someone whom they know to be vulnerable, and for whom they have a responsibility. The decision-making processes are complex, and achieving the appropriate balance between rights and risks can be extremely difficult.

This chapter expores the concepts of rights, responsibilities, and risk and how they can be balanced in situations that arise every day in care homes. It specifically focuses on how nurses can help to promote and facilitate genuine choices for older people that maintain their rights, even when are physically frail or cognitively impaired. It also highlights key issues regarding risk management. The chapter offers some case study examples, and practical ideas of how nurses can work with older people in mutual respect and partnership, towards choice, healthy risk-taking and the promotion of rights for all.

The concepts of rights, responsibilities and risk

Rights

The concept of rights is complex. It implies entitlements which should morally, ethically or legally, or fairly belong to an individual. Yet few rights are either absolute or timeless, and it could be argued that rights only exist insofar as they are granted by those around us. Rights, therefore, exist in a relationship between individuals, or an individual and a community of people, and relate to the concept of responsibility (Norman, 1980). Individuals may choose to exercise their rights but, if physical or mental frailty impairs this process, it may be appropriate for others to assist. The concept of rights thus links to the concepts of need, and dependence/independence.

A person's legal rights are not affected by moving into a care home. Furthermore there is no assumption in law that, by choosing or agreeing to move into a home, a person has voluntarily surrendered his/her rights. In addition, rights of citizenship should not be affected when a person moves into a care home in that he/she should enjoy the same liberty granted to other adult citizens to control personal affairs, finances and daily activities.

The Royal College of Nursing and British Medical Association state:

> Older people have the same rights to services, and to health care in particular, as do other members of society. We know that the life of an older person is just as valuable as that of a younger individual, and judgements about the quality of that life are the sole prerogative of the person living it. We know there is no justification for dismissing these people as a burden, or for judging the value of life solely on the basis of age. Yet, despite these facts, the rights of older people are often ignored, and the ability of these people to dictate the quality of their life is often overlooked by well-intentioned individuals.
>
> (British Medical Association and
> Royal College of Nursing, 1995)

Responsibilities

Under the law, each person has responsibility for him/herself, unless he/she is mentally ill in a manner which brings him/her within the scope of mental health legislation (Counsel and Care, 1992a).

Responsibilities in care homes are multiple. Each person in a home has some responsibility for the safety and well-being of others and, in particular, nurses have responsibility to care for people who are dependent on them (see Chapter 3: Professional Nursing Issues). However, Counsel and Care (1992a) argue that this responsibility is not necessarily to prevent all harm, but to balance responsible caring with risk-taking in order to allow for individual freedom.

The more rights and freedoms that exist in a home, the greater the risks.

Risk

Risk can be defined as the possibility of incurring misfortune, loss, or danger. Risk can also be viewed as an element of life which adds sparkle and, without which, life would be impoverished (Counsel and Care, 1992a).

In care homes, every action and circumstance involves danger of some kind. As Norman (1987) argues, 'there is no drug without side-effects, no piece of routine which does not limit choice, no movement which could not cause an accident, and no professional decision which could not be mistaken'. It is important that nurses are aware of potential risks to people who are physically or mentally vulnerable, and for whom they have a responsibility. The challenge is to minimise undue risk without infringing on an individual's rights or choices.

Maintaining rights in care homes

The rights of older people are sometimes eroded, without the realisation that this is happening. Consider these examples:

- *On Miss A's case notes her first names are Eileen Elsie. Staff call her Eileen. In fact she has never used these names, being known in her family as 'Billy' and would rather be called 'Miss A' by the staff. (Erosion of the right to be addressed as you wish.)*
- *Mrs B has asked if the staff will knock on her bedroom door before entering. They now remember to knock but don't wait for an answer. (Erosion of the right to control a personal space and to resist intrusion.)*
- *Mr C's wife can only visit on a Sunday. They want to spend time alone in his room but staff like to make sure they're alright by periodically looking through the glass panel in the door. (Erosion of the right to privacy and choice of company.)*

In order to prevent rights being eroded, a key starting point is the facilitation of choice.

Choice

Many homes aim to offer older people the maxium choice possible but, in reality, the choices may be limited. One survey asked a group of older people attending a day hospital what choices and facilities they would want when they moved into a home. The study then interviewed a second group of older people living in care homes to ascertain what facilities they had.

- 90% of those not yet in homes said they would want control over their own money. 38% of those in homes had some control.
- 67% of day hospital attenders said they would want a choice of food. 35% of those living in homes had this choice.
- 73% in the day hospital said they would want to choose menus in advance. 36% of people in homes could do so.
- 81% of those not yet in homes said they would want a choice of when to get up in the morning. 52% of older people in homes had this choice.

(Counsel and Care, 1992b)

Real choice implies a genuine selection from a range of alternatives. It also implies that choices will be respected, and that the person choosing will thus have control over how they live their lives. Many care homes offer as many choices as they can but, if residents then select alternatives that make staff feel uncomfortable (such as not eating, washing, or getting out of bed), staff often try to persuade the resident to change his/her mind, or even override the decision for their own, or organisational, goals. The reaction of staff in these circumstances can indicate the location of the real power and control in the home. Many care plans in homes also indicate the locus of real power by stating that the nurses will 'give Mrs. D a choice of food' or 'allow Mr. E to get up when he wants'. As McCormack (1994) says 'Choice is not ours to give or allow, but it is ours to promote and facilitate'.

Promoting and facilitating real choice for older people in homes not only prevents erosion of their rights, but also helps them to have control over their lives. Research has demonstrated that choice and control contribute to positive health outcomes, and enhance both quality and quantity of life (Rodin, 1986, 1989; Aasen, 1982; Ryden, 1984; Phillips, 1986). Loss of control is associated with ill health, psychological distress, and increased mortality (Robertson, 1986; Abrahamson, Seligman and Teasdale, 1978).

Choices which may be detrimental to health

Some of the most difficult decisions arise when older people make choices which nurses feel would put them at risk, would be detrimental to their health, or would go against medical or nursing advice. The following examples illustrate key issues, which are discussed later in the chapter:

- *Mrs F had a stroke recently and her speech is severely impaired. Every time her leg ulcer is treated, she shouts and pushes the nurses away. They are unable to understand what she is saying.*
- *Mr G has Parkinson's disease. His tremors have recently become much worse and he is now refusing to eat.*
- *Mrs H has become mentally confused over the past day or so. She is now refusing all medication, including her thyroxine tablets.*
- *Mrs I had advanced dementia and walks around for most of the day. In the late afternoon she oftens wants to go out of the home.*

These situations are not straightforward but, in each situation, there is potential for the rights and choices of the older person to be eroded.

How rights can become eroded and choices overriden

When nurses are meeting these kinds of situations, there are influences bearing on them. It is important to be aware of these, particularly when deciding to override a person's choice, or making a decision for him or her.

- Nurses know that the person is vulnerable, and that they have a duty to protect, support and care for them. This can lead to an emphasis on protecting.
- Because the older person is, to a degree, dependent on the nurse, the balance of power in the relationship is unequal. In fact nurses often unintentionally reinforce this power balance in many aspects of their day to day work, including controlling language (Lanceley, 1985).
- Health care professionals generally expect people who are ill, and dependent upon them, to comply with their advice. In fact, it is often when patients do not comply that their mental competence is first questioned.
- People who are dependent and disempowered may tend to comply without questioning.
- Health professionals make decisions based on their own personal values. These may include a whole range of values about ways of living, ways of dying, the importance of religion, or the appropriateness of sex in older age. The values of the health professional may be totally different to those of the older person, and there may thus be covert pressure on the resident.
- Nurses, particularly in continuing care settings and care homes, will often consult the resident's family on a decision, particularly when the family is seen as the customer of the service (Heath, 1994). The values of family members may be different to those of the older person, particularly with regard to risk-taking and, again, there is pressure on the resident to conform to the wishes of others.

In order to help older people in care homes retain their rights and exercise their choices, nurses should consider their personal values, the values of the organisation within which they work, and their legal and professional responsibilities.

Considering personal values

Personal values are formed as a result of multiple influences.

Cultural and societal values: How older people are viewed by both society and nurses has been discussed in volumes of literature (such as Thompson, 1991; Fielding, 1986). In practice, whether a nurse considers an older person to be a repository of life experience and wisdom and a valuable member of society, or alternatively a weakened, non-productive, burden on society, will influence how actively he/she seeks the older person's choices.

Individual and generational experiences: Most nurses are in the younger and middle-aged groups. This may influence their expectations of how older people, and specifically older people in care homes, behave. If an older person adamantly asserts her rights, contrary to the expectations of the staff, the resident's behaviour may be considered eccentric, or worse as a manifestation of mental impairment.

Beliefs about the nurse–older person (patient) relationship: A fundamental tenet of many nurses is that they care for 'their' patients, as if they have some ownership. This caring can derive from a need to nurture, and has been related to fundamental ethical principles such as beneficence, which loosely means the promotion of the well-being of another (Singleton and McLaren, 1995). However if, by promoting beneficence, the nurse overrides the person's rights to self-determination, this becomes paternalism.

Paternalism is doing what is believed to be in the person's interests without regard to, or by overriding, that person's wishes. Paternalism has been rife throughout health care for many decades, and it is not an appropriate principle upon which to base the care of older people.

An ethical principle more appropriate for the care of older people in communal homes is that of autonomy. This has been defined as 'the capacity to think, decide, and act on the basis of such thought and decision freely and independently' (Gillon, 1990).

Considering the values of the organisation, and the way it operates

In every organisation there are distinct pressures. In recent times public awareness of inadequate care in homes has been raised by reporters with hidden cameras, the work of Action on Elder Abuse, and the UKCC report of professional conduct hearings of nursing home nurses (UKCC, 1994). Many home managers have felt pressured into making detailed statements on what is, or is not, acceptable practice in their homes. This could have the effect of limiting flexible practices, and thus limiting resident freedom.

Some home owners would suggest that, particularly if staffing levels are low, it is impossible not to restrict freedom in some ways. However, it is important that all regimes which potentially restrict freedom are kept under review in order that the organisational goals of the home do not override individual rights. It is essential also that residents are encouraged to express their wishes and their views on the running of their home. If decisions are always made on behalf of residents, these people can easily succumb to the habit of acquiescence. This cycle of disempowerment is well-documented, and results in the resident's 'learned helplessness' (Robertson, 1986).

Considering legal responsibilities

Nurses have various legal responsibilities which relate to promoting the rights of their patients. These are discussed fully in other texts (Caulfield, 1995; Tingle and Cribb, 1995).

If individuals are able to understand, make and express a choice then, in the majority of circumstances, the nurse must support this. However, difficulties arise if it is unclear as to whether the individual can understand, make or express a choice, as in some of the examples described earlier. A key concept in these circumstances is that of consent, and particularly in terms of giving consent to treatment. Consent can be defined as the 'voluntary and continuing permission of the patient to·receive a particular treatment, based on adequate knowledge of the purpose, nature, likely effects and risks of that treatment, including the likelihood of its success and any alternatives to it. Permission given under any unfair or undue pressure is not consent' (Department of Health, Welsh Office, 1993).

Under the law, a key aspect of obtaining valid consent is the ability, 'capacity' or mental 'competence' of an individual to give consent. The BMA and the Law Society guidance suggests that, in order to have capacity, the person must be able to:

- understand, in broad terms and simple language, what the treatment is, its purpose and nature, and why the treatment is being proposed for him or her,
- understand its principal benefits, risks and alternatives,
- understand, in broad terms, the consequences of not receiving the proposed treatment,
- possess the capacity to make a choice free from pressure, and
- retain the information long enough for an effective decision.

Competent adults have a clear right to refuse treatment for reasons which are 'rational, irrational or for no reason' (British Medical Association and Royal College of Nursing, 1995).

> *If Mrs F meets the above criteria, and is therefore deemed to be mentally 'competent' to refuse the treatment of her leg ulcer, then this is her right.*

Mental capacity or 'competence' to consent to care is less clear cut. Fundamental care can be defined as assisting people to do those things which they would normally do for themselves if they were able, such as keeping themselves warm, dry, clean and comfortable.

> *Thus, if Mr G. is deemed to be 'competent' then he can refuse to accept fundamental care, or indeed any form of physical contact, and it would be both unethical and illegal to force this upon him, and forcibly feed him.*
>
> (British Medical Association and
> Royal College of Nursing, 1995)

However, when a person is considered unable to have the capacity to consent to, or refuse, fundamental care, the Law Commission and the BMA state that 'anyone who has care of an incapacitated person (or has reasonable grounds for believing a person in his or her care to be incapacitated) may do what is reasonable in all the circumstances to care for that person and to safeguard and promote his or her welfare' (English Law Commission, 1993).

Considering professional responsibilities

The UKCC Code of Conduct (1992) states that a registered nurse should 'act always in such a manner as to promote and safeguard the interests and wellbeing of patients and clients'. It would seem consistent with the spirit of the code that the nurse should act always to preserve the person's rights and autonomy and, when the person does not have the 'capacity' to consent, to try, as far as possible, to do what that person would want.

Assessment

Before a decision can be made on an individual older person's mental 'capacity' to consent to, or refuse, care or treatment, a thorough and skillful assessment needs to be made. Families and friends of the older person can provide significant information, and the assessment should be agreed by a team including the nurses, GP, and other other professional involved in the person's care such as a physiotherapist, speech therapist or social worker.

It is important to remember that very few people are totally incapable of making any decision.

Physically frail people, and particularly those with communication difficulties, may find it extremely difficult to express their choices coherently, but this does not mean that they are unable to make choices.

> *In people who have had strokes, such as Mrs F, there may also be perceptual and other neurological changes which mean that they say 'yes' when they mean 'no', or move to the left when they are trying to move to the right.*

Difficulty in expressing choices *does not* equate to mental incapacity. Offered adequate time and appropriate communication methods, these people can be helped to express their wishes, and their rights thus preserved.

When assessing an older person's 'capacity' to make a decision, or consent to treatment, it is important to remember that, particularly in mental frailty, capacity can change according to the environment, the people around, the time of the day, physiological status, or medication reactions. Competence to make decisions can therefore be difficult to establish. Partial capacity is not the same as 'capacity' or 'incapacity' and, in these situations, competence is a relative, rather than an absolute state.

> *When assessing Mrs H, who is refusing her medication, the nurse should try to identify the reason. There may be an underlying physiological change (such as dehydration) or toxin accumulation (from infection or constipation) that is causing an acute/toxic confusional state. If treated, the person's usual mental state will return. It is thus important to identify all physiological influences on the person's mental state, and treat them. Other physical influences include pain and fatigue.*

If a person refuses treatment or care, it is also helpful to identify any psychological influences on this decision.

For example is Mr G. refusing to eat because he is reacting to his current state of ill health or disability? Is he depressed, feeling powerless, or even losing the will to continue living?

It is important to offer choices to all residents as, even if they are unable to make decisions on all aspects of life, they will be able to make some choices. For example, a person with advanced dementia may not be deemed legally 'competent' to consent to treatment but, given a selection of clothes or food, he/she will often be able to make a choice.

Thus 'incompetency' in one area of decision-making does not necessarily mean incompetence in another, and assessment of capacity must be made on a decision-specific basis.

Facilitating choice in day-to-day situations

There are many skills and techniques that nurses can use to promote and facilitate the expression of choice. These may be particularly helpful when working with people who are mentally frail. Connecting with the person's life history is important. If the nurse understands how the person has lived, it is easier for her/him to know how the person would want to live. By undertaking biographical assessment (Schofield, 1994) and compiling a values history, the nurse can better understand any significant life experiences (e.g. bereavements) and what is important to that person (such as work or prayer). This is particularly important for people from varying cultures or religious sects, and for those who speak different languages. Much of this information can be gained through daily interactions with the older person.

Nurses use a range of skills in building relationships, communicating and supporting (see Chapter 10: Communications).

When there are decisions to be made, and the person is mentally frail, various techniques can be used:

- The decision can be delayed until an optimum time arises, such as a lucid phase, or a relative's visit.
- Time should be allowed for the decision-making
- Written information can help the person to reflect on the issues in his/her own time. It can also help to reinforce the benefits and risks of a situation.

However mentally frail the older person, the nurse should aim to maintain maximum autonomy and choice in as many aspects of daily life as possible, e.g. what time to get up, what to eat, what to wear. This is particularly important in order that the older person's capacity for, and interest in, decision-making is preserved.

Success breeds success. In order to maintain self-respect and self-esteem, it is important to reinforce successful choices and behaviours, taking care not to patronise or infantilise the older person. It is also important to prevent the person from failing, whenever this is possible (Kitwood, 1993). For someone with severe cognitive impairment, it may be appropriate to limit the choices to help prevent failure. For example, offering food appropriate for the culture and time of day, or clothes appropriate for the weather. It may sometimes be appropriate to guide the choices.

> *For example, as Mrs I is wanting to go outside, the nurse could say 'Here's your coat Mrs I – it's bitterly cold out today'. If Mrs I refuses this suggestion, the nurse could accept Mrs I's decision, then return within a short time and repeat the original request, or divert Mrs I's attention and repeat the request once she has forgotten the original conversation.*

Caplan (1985) refers to 'assisted' decision-making as maximising capacity, taking time and effort to support decision-making, rather than remove the potential for capacity.

Acting in 'best interests'

If, after thorough assessment, a person is deemed to have lost the 'capacity' to consent to, or refuse, treatment, health professionals must then act in the person's best interests (Re F, 1990). There is no clear test for generally determining what course of action would be in a person's best interests, but there are principles:

- Consult with other professionals. A shared decision is preferable to a single professional decision being substituted for that of the older person (Kapp, 1988).
- Consult with relatives and those close to the older person, as they probably have valuable insight into what the individual would want. However, remember that *in law, no person can give consent to treatment on behalf of another*. Relatives should therefore not be asked to sign consent forms. (The Law Commission is currently exploring possibilities for changing this law.)
- If the person is temporarily incapacitated, postpone the decision.
- If treatment is to safeguard life, health or wellbeing, then health professionals may be legally bound to give treatment without consent.

> *If, after thorough assessment, it was decided that, because of her confused state, Mrs H had temporarily lost the 'capacity' to consent, but needed the thyroxine to maintain her health, staff could decide they had a legal obligation to administer treatment.*

However, treatment should not be given where there is convincing evidence that the patient would have withheld consent (for example the administration of a blood transfusion to a devout Jehovah's Witness).

- Recognise that active treatment may not always be the best course of action for the person, e.g. chemotherapy in terminal cancer.
- Individuals who do not overtly object to preventative health measures, such as breast or prostatic screening, should not be deprived of the potential benefits.

- People who lack capacity to give consent may be treated under the Mental Health Act 1983, provided that they fall within the remit of the relevant section.
- Best efforts should be made to establish and adhere to the patient's known views and preferences.

In care homes nurses establish close relationships with the residents. They may assume that they understand the person's values and can predict what decisions they might make. Although these judgements may be sound, the above points should be considered before assumptions are made.

Advocacy

Nurses often act as advocates for people in their care who are unable to represent their own interests, and try to represent these interests as faithfully as possible. Citizen advocacy schemes are being developed around the country by organisations such as Age Concern, and these may be available to care homes. Citizen advocates have no close association with either the older person or the care providers, and offer their services without prior influence, interest or prejudice. When establishing advocacy, it is important that the process be regulated, in particular where confidentiality is concerned. It is also important to clearly establish on whose authority the advocate is acting.

The Centre for Policy on Ageing has now developed a code of practice for citizen advocacy projects with older people, and is recommending that recognised regulation be established in this area (Dunning, 1995).

Risk assessment and risk management

Care homes are increasingly developing risk assessment and risk management policies and protocols. Residents and their families can be involved in these developments. In particular, the staff need to understand and own the policies. Care homes are very individual in terms of their design (e.g. steep stairs), their situations (e.g. adjacent to a busy road), their residents and their staffing levels and skill mixes. All of these factors are relevant in policy development.

Policies and protocols should contain explicit statements that some degree of risk is intrinsic to the human experience and in the interests of the expression of human rights, liberties and freedoms. Unpredicted outcomes are not necessarily a failure of the home or of individuals, provided that all reasonable efforts have been made to facilitate individual rights and choices, while minimising unacceptable risks. Protocols should include some guidance for staff when residents appear to be endangering themselves, fellow residents or staff. Adequately skilled staff and appropriate training are essential in these circumstances.

Potential residents and their families can be made aware of the home's risk assessment and management policies before the older person moves in. This can be an opportunity for discussing potential risks (that no home can be a totally safe environment), and obtaining views on risks.

Counsel and Care (1992a) suggest that areas within which risk-taking assessment could be conducted include:

- privacy and use of rooms and bedroom,
- going out alone,
- visitors,
- visiting outside the home, to clubs, pubs or religious centres,
- engaging in recreational and leisure pursuits,
- carrying identification (photographs),
- medication,
- consulting a doctor or other specialist,
- diet and food issues,
- preparing food, using kettles and other appliances,
- clothes and laundry,
- financial affairs,
- pattern of the day, and
- any agreed restriction on choice of activities.

In reaching decisions about risk, the key input is the view of the older person. Relatives should also be consulted, but the older person's view should not be subjugated to theirs. The risk should be identified and the gains listed (such as feeling of control, personal fulfilment) alongside the potential losses (such as physical danger). The gains and losses can then be considered alongside the magnitude of each (for example the loss of a small amount of money, or a life-threatening circumstance). The likelihood of the occurrence of the losses or harm can then be placed into the balance and, finally, alternatives to the same end can be considered.

For people who are not able to make and express 'competent' (in the legal sense) choices, risk assessment and risk-taking are less straight-forward.

> In the case of Mrs I, who had advanced dementia, and often wants to walk out of the home, a thorough and skilled assessment needs to be undertaken. During this assessment, a relative explains that Mrs I's son died in the war but, because she believes he is coming home, she wants to meet him at the railway station. A risk assessment would balance potential gains from helping Mrs I go to out (such as her peace of mind) alongside the potential risks (from busy roads, or her getting lost), the magnitude of each, and the likelihood of the danger. A variety of strategies could be used for facilitate her wishes, such as someone accompanying her to the station, and also to help meet her need to walk around the home (see Chapter 7: Home Life and Chapter 11: Mental Health).

There is one circumstance in which the needs of the individual may be of secondary priority, and that is where the choice of that individual places at risk the safety or welfare of other residents in the home or the local community. It may well be that, in these circumstances, the well-being of the greater number of people takes precedence.

In both risk assessment and risk management, it is vital that staff are adequately trained. For example, if the rights of residents are to be preserved, nurses need skills to elicit and interpret the older person's wishes. Education can also promote and support professional confidence by helping nurses to be aware of all the implications of their actions. This is particularly important when nurses are exercising judgements which involve risk-taking, and which could result in retrospective recriminations should accidents occur.

Documentation

It is important that key elements of the risk assessment are agreed and documented for each older person. The risk can be recorded on each person's care, or daily living, plan, including details of the aims of the risk or care strategy, how the aims are to be achieved, and specific abilities or barriers for the older person in achieving the aims. They may contain contracts relevant to specific risks, in which the older person specifies that, despite any risks, he/she wishes to undertake a particular activity. Care plans, or daily living plans, should be signed and dated, with appropriate review periods. Information can be accessible to residents and staff, but confidentiality to non-involved persons should be borne in mind. Care plans, or daily living plans, should be operational documents that are used and updated appropriately. Above all, care plans should be individual, focusing on the wishes and needs of the older person.

Openness – the home in the community

One of the problems identified in the UKCC (1994) report into professional misconduct in nursing homes identified that, where there was a closed environment, with few changes of staff and residents and few visitors from outside, potentially harmful practices were more likely to develop. One safeguard against institutional practices is to encourage the home to be a part of the local community. Relatives and friends of the residents, but also groups or individuals from churches or religious centres, voluntary groups, or schools, can be encouraged to visit. Additionally, the residents should be encouraged to maintain their personal links in the community (see Chapter 7: Home Life).

In many areas, homes have formed into groups which act as peer support systems through which staff can share their concerns and their ideas for good practice. Homes can set up discussion groups or joint training programmes specifically for staff in that sector. Local inspectors and registration officers can be valuable advisers, not only on registration requirements, but also on good practice.

Care homes can also offer valuable experiences to new student nurses, who will increasingly be working in care homes when they qualify. The students' fresh perspectives can also be valuable to staff, and can bring new ideas and ways of working.

Information should be offered to residents and prospective residents about their rights and responsibilities, the polices of the home on risk, and complaints procedures. In fact, the perspectives of the residents and their families can make valuable contributions to the development and revision of these policies. Resident and family contributions to rights and risks policies help to ensure that they are user-friendly and are workable in practice. The involvement also helps residents and families to understand the intricacies of individual situations, and to feel a sense of ownership.

Conclusions

Maintaining a balance between rights, risks and responsibilities is a highly complex and challenging aspect of nursing older people within care homes. This chapter has reviewed key ethical, legal and professional perspectives on the subject, and has offered some guidelines for nurses in their day-to-day work with older people. A starting point of good practice is to recognise the rights and responsibilities of all those who live and work in the home, alongside the need to take risks. Practices should encourage openness, consultation and the empowerment of individuals. Thorough and ongoing assessment is fundamental, as are staff training, and documentation. Life in care homes will never be totally free of risk. The challenge is to create a culture within which staff can skilfully, professionally and safely take decisions that will promote rights, and encourage responsible risk-taking. 'If this seems a tentative conclusion, this is a measure of the complexity of the situation and of the uncertainty with which our society currently approaches the issue' (Counsel and Care, 1992a).

Useful contacts

Action on Elder Abuse, Astral House, 1268 London Road, London SW16 4ER.
Age Concern England, Astral House, 1268 London Road, London SW16 4ER.
Age Concern Northern Ireland, 3 Lower Crescent, Belfast BT7 1NR.
Age Concern Scotland, 54a Fountainbridge, Edinburgh EH3 9PT.
Age Concern Wales, 4th Floor, 1 Cathedral Road, Cardiff CF1 9SD.
Counsel and Care, Twyman House, 16 Bonny Street, London NW1 9PG.

References

Aasen, N. (1982) Interventions to facilitate personal control. *Journal of Gerontological Nursing*, **13**, 6, 21–28.
Abrahamson, L.Y., Seligman, M.E.P. and Teasdale, J.D. (1978) Learned helplessness. *Journal of Abnormal Psychology*, **87**, 1, 49–74.

British Medical Association and Royal College of Nursing (1995) *The Older Person: Consent and Care.* London: British Medical Assocation.

Caplan, A.L. (1985) Let wisdom find a way. *Generations,* **19**, 10–14.

Caulfield, H. (1995) Legal Aspects. In H.B.M. Heath (ed.) *Foundations in Nursing Theory and Practice.* London: Mosby.

Counsel and Care (1992a) What if They Hurt Themselves: A discussion document on the uses and abuses of restraint in residential care and nursing homes for older people. London: Counsel and Care.

Counsel and Care (1992b) From Home to a Home: A study of older people's hopes, expectations and experiences of residential care. London: Counsel and Care.

Counsel and Care (1993) The Right to Take Risks: Model policies, guidance to staff and training material on restraint and risk taking in residential care and nursing homes for older people. London: Counsel and Care.

Department of Health Welsh Office (1993) Code of Practice, Mental Health Act 1983. London: Department of Health.

Dunning, A. (1995) Citizen Advocacy with Older People: A Code of Good Practice. London: Centre for Policy on Ageing.

English Law Commission (1993) Mentally Incapacitated Adults and Decison-Making: A New Jurisdiction. London: English Law Commission.

Fielding, P. (1986) Attitudes revisited. London: Royal College of Nursing.

Gillon, R. (1990) *Philosophical Medical Ethics.* Chichester: John Wiley.

Heath, H. (1994) Sexuality in later life: How nurses in nursing homes and continuing care settings facilitate the expression of sexuality by older residents. Unpublished MSc thesis, University of Surrey.

Kapp, M.B. (1988) Forcing services on at-risk older adults: when doing good is not so good. *Social Work in Health Care,* **13**, 4, 1–13.

Kitwood, T. (1993) Towards a theory of dementia care: the interpersonal process. *Ageing and Society,* **13**, 51–67.

Lanceley, A. (1985) Use of controlling language in the rehabilitation of the eldery. *Journal of Advanced Nursing,* **10**, 125–135.

McCormack, B. (1994) The Professional Aspects of Choice (paper presented at conference, Whose Choice is it Anyway? Royal College of Nursing Association for the Care of Elderly People, Exeter University).

Norman, A. (1987) Risk or restraint? *Nursing Times,* **83**, 30, 31.

Norman, A. (1980) Rights and risk: A discussion document in civil liberty in old age. London: National Corporation for the Care of Old People.

Phillips, D. (1986) Assessing dependency in old people's homes: Problems of purpose and method. Part 1: Issues in policy utilisation. *Social Services Research,* **6**, 23–44.

Phillips, D. (1986) Assessing dependency in old people's homes: Problems of purpose and method. Part 2: Creating dependency measures. *Social Services Research,* **7**, 30–46.

Re, F. (1990) 2 AC 1. (Clarification of the law on treatment of incapacitated patients).

Robertson, I. (1986) Learned helplessness. *Nursing Times* **82**(51), 28–29.

Rodin, J. (1986) Ageing and health: effects on the sense of control. *Science*, **233**, 1271.

Rodin, J. (1989) Sense of control: Potentials for intervention, Annals, Advance in Applied Psychology, **503**, May.

Ryden, M.B. (1984) Morale and perceived control in the institutionalised elderly. *Nursing Research*, **33**, 3, 130–136.

Schofield, I. (1994) Using a historical approach to care. *Elderly Care*, **6**, 6, 14–15.

Singleton, J. and McLaren, S. (1995) *Ethical Foundations of Health Care: Responsibilities in Decision Making*. London: Mosby.

Thompson, H. (1991) Attitudes to old people: a review, Part 1. *Nursing Standard*, **5**, 30, 33–36.

Thompson, H. (1991) Attitudes to old people: a review, Part 2. *Nursing Standard*, **5**, 31, 33–35.

Tingle, J. and Cribb, A. (1995) *Nursing Law and Ethics*. Oxford: Blackwell Science Ltd.

United Kingdom Central Council for Nursing, Midwifery and Health Visiting (1994) Professional Conduct – Occasional Report on Standards of Nursing in Nursing Homes. London: UKCC.

United Kingdom Central Council for Nursing, Midwifery and Health Visiting (1992) Code of Professional Conduct. London: UKCC.

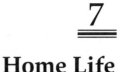

7

Home Life

Maria Scurfield

Introduction

As with any age group, older people have a right to make decisions and have choices about where they want to live and about the types of care they receive. Although, in most situations, older people are able to make a choice regarding their home, the choice to enter a nursing home is seldom planned by the resident. However, the final decision to enter should be personal.

The importance of the environment within the care home setting cannot be over-emphasised. If we consider what home means to us, we see that it is an expression of our individuality. Our home expresses a wealth of information about our preferences, personalities, attitudes and lifestyles (Eliopoulos, 1993).

Garrett (1991) states that a home fulfils many needs; it is a place of shelter and security, in which there is a sense of belonging and mastery, which allows the person to be him or herself and which reinforces (by the presence of significant personal items) their life experience and identity.

Relocation from home to a care home setting presents a radical change for older people. As individuals we all use our day and night hours differently. Sleep patterns, work patterns and recreation patterns vary considerably. A continuing care setting is a community with a wide variety of personalities and characters, as in any other community. Communal life places certain limitations on responding to each individual's lifestyle.

This chapter will explore how the care home environment can be managed to enhance opportunities to create a homely environment that promotes individualised care. Suggestions of positive strategies to create opportunities to balance the older person's lifestyle within the care home setting will be explored.

Principles of good practice

- Recognition of individuality of the older person.
- Respect for each individual's privacy and personal territory.
- Older people are consulted and involved in their personal care.
- Each individual is allowed to do things at his or her own pace and when he or she wishes.

- Opportunities are provided to engage residents in activities of their own choice.
- Cultural, sexual and religious needs are respected.
- Each older person is given maximum control and choice over his or her lifestyle within the home.
- Opportunities are provided for inclusion of the individual's personal possessions.
- Opportunities are provided for individuals to continue their pre-home lifestyle within the home and the local community.
- Older persons' families and friends are encouraged to visit and contribute to their relatives' care.
- Individuals are encouraged to discuss concerns about their care.
- Opportunities are provided for ongoing training and support for professional and personal development of staff.

Environmental considerations

Care home settings are unable to provide the same gratification as the older person's own home, but the environment can be enhanced by the physical surroundings and, more importantly, by the positive care-giving attitudes of the nursing staff. This enhances the opportunities to establish an individual, active lifestyle within the care home setting.

Many older people have negative images of themselves; this can be especially so in circumstances when the older person becomes more dependent on others because of illness, impairment or disability.

There is a danger that the care home setting may disempower the older person. The care home environment can strive to empower older people by supporting their independence, their right to freedom of choice, and their right to be involved in decisions about their care. The environment should promote the continued development of the older person. Old age should not be viewed as a negative experience that is linked with general decline. Indeed, old age should be viewed as a time when happiness, fulfilment, health and new learning are achievable (Royal College of Nursing, 1993).

Physical environment

Due to the sensory changes associated with ageing, older people have special needs in relation to the environment. Environmental needs are also created by conditions such as osteoporosis, arthritis or cognitive impairment. Nurses are able to manipulate aspects of the environment to compensate for older persons' limitations, and to enhance their functioning.

The environment should have aids, equipment and furniture such as, signs, ramps, wide toilets, raised toilet seats, hand rails, etc. These resources enable older people to have some control over their movement and daily activities. However, such equipment can create a 'clinical' impression, and the environment is less likely to look homely. Nurses must recognise that the most important aspect of a 'homely' environment is created by enhancing opportunities for each older person to follow the lifestyle that either they are used to, or that they desire.

Lighting

Visual and colour environment is particularly important for older people as, with ageing, depth perception tends to weaken, rapid adaptation between light and dark becomes more difficult, and colour discrimination, particularly between blues and greens, becomes less effective (Garland, 1991).

Lighting is an important aspect of a care home setting for older people. Eliopoulos, (1993) suggests that light has several abilities apart from illuminating an area for better visibility. Lighting can affect the person's orientation, for example the older person may lose his or her sense of time if they are in a room that is either constantly lightened or darkened for long periods. Lighting also affects a person's functioning. For example, the older person may interact and engage in activities more in a brightly lighted area. The opposite may happen if the older person sits in a dim room. Lighting also affects a person's mood and behaviour. For example, blinking psychedelic lights can cause the older person to become restless.

Due to age-related physical changes in the eye, the levels of illumination required by an older person is increased (Yurick, Spier, Robb and Ebert, 1989). Glare and eye strain should be avoided, therefore bright and fluorescent lights are undesirable. Diffuse lighting sources are more appropriate. It is important that switches are easily accessible and placed in areas that are potentially dangerous for example, doorways, halls and stairways. Lighting is also important at night so that the older person can travel to the toilet and bathroom safely.

Contrast and colour

Poor use of contrast and colour in care home settings for older people is not acceptable. Invisible glass doors and white electric switches against white walls do not promote safety, well-being or independence. Safety and independence can be increased by use of contrasting colours to enhance the visibility of objects.

Light-coloured plates can be placed on dark tables or dark coloured plates can be placed on a white surface. Cullinan (1991) suggests that a coloured object on a white surface is preferable to a white object on a dark surface (bright surfaces reflect 70 to 80 per cent of the light falling on it, a dark one not more than 20 per cent).

Stairs often prove difficult for older people who have visual impairment. The use of a contrasting colour on the edge of each step will enhance the older person's ability to manage the steps. In many care home areas, colours are used to define different areas. To help promote memory and orientation, colour coding is often used to identify individual's bedrooms, or facilities such as the bathrooms or toilets.

Research into types of colour to stimulate moods and activity has also been conducted. Pale clear, blues and greens provide a relaxing, stimulating atmosphere; yellows are cheerful, and a place with touches of bright red encourage activity (Worsley, 1992).

Carpets and furniture

A careful choice of floor covering can promote a homely atmosphere within the care home setting. Carpets also provide a better buffer against falls than linoleum and, as older people are at risk of fractures due to falls, carpeting should be a major consideration.

The choice of furniture is also an important factor when attempting to create a homely environment and maintaining the older person's independence. A care home setting that has individual bedrooms has much more scope for personal choices in furniture for the room. Older people can be given scope to furnish their bedrooms with their own furniture and memorabilia. If the care home setting only provides dormitory-style bedrooms, it is important that nurses create adequate space and privacy between each person's bed; for example, locks on cupboards and doors could enhance privacy. Again, older people should be encouraged to bring in their own memorabilia. Many care homes encourage residents to bring in their own television, and, in some homes, telephones are installed into bedrooms. This obviously enhances choice and promotes a sense of control and freedom for the older person.

Chairs are possibly the most important items of furniture within a care home. This is because so much of the older person's time is spent in them. Well-designed chairs are vital to the older person's independence and quality of life. People experience difficulty in getting out of a chair that is too low or has no arms.

One of the most disheartening features of many care home settings is the lounge where chairs are arranged around the walls. This type of arrangement discourages interaction and conversation between older people. Older people with sensory impairment may soon become disorientated and withdrawn if attempts to enhance communication are not provided.

If space is very limited then it may be very difficult to arrange chairs any other way. A dilemma may occur between encouraging social interaction between older people and protecting their privacy.

Psycho-social considerations

By far the most important aspects of creating a homely environment are the attitudes of the staff towards older people, and their ability to maintain the older person's pre-home lifestyle. An environment that is beautifully decorated means little when individuality, respect and sensitivity are not present.

Much can be learned by the nurse about the older person's lifestyle, his or her likes and dislikes, and individual needs. Visiting the older person in his or her own home prior to admission into the care home setting provides excellent opportunities for the nurse to assess the person's lifestyle and needs. It also provides the opportunity to establish a relationship with the older person, which may make the move seem less threatening. Assessment of the older person's lifestyle and activities of daily living should be undertaken in an informal and relaxed manner. Older people will respond more openly to a nurse who shows interest and concern.

Assessment of the older person

While visiting prior to admission, the nurses can build up a profile of the older person. Information may include the person's full name and preference of title; gender; race; name of spouse or partner, family members and contact person; name and location of church or religious centre, etc.

Assessment of the older person's lifestyle should follow a typical day from the time the person gets up until the time he or she retires to bed. Information may include the following: sleep patterns, variations and quality of sleep; diet and fluid intake in a 24 hour period and how many times a day do they eat; preferences, strengths and ability to accomplish activities of daily living; life events and activities that give the person a sense of identity; family and friends' involvement, and social and leisure activities.

A change in home is a major life event and the impact it can have on the older person should not be underestimated. If the move is as a result of changes, for example retirement, ill health, or death of a spouse and particularly if the older person has little choice but to move, the effect of such changes may prove fatal (Garrett, 1991). Continuity of the older person's pre-home lifestyle is therefore extremely important.

Moving into the home

Settling into a care home requires thought, planning, time and space. Making advanced visits to the home will help the older person to decide on the move, how this might best be accomplished, and what he or she wishes to bring into the home by way of personal belongings. Bringing furniture and significant possessions will enhance the older person's feelings of ownership in the new environment.

Care staff can lessen the trauma of the move by demonstrating sensitivity to the feelings of the older person, and ensuring that the new resident is fully introduced to the care staff and the new environment.

Continuity of lifestyle

When an older person moves into a care home, it is important that every effort is made to ensure that their lifestyle and social contacts continue. A biographical assessment is one way of establishing the priorities and significant experiences of an older person (Schofield, 1994). Using biographies, and approaches such as reminiscence and life review, can be extremely effective in easing the transition from home to the care home, and in helping the older person adjust to his or her new situation in life (see Chapter 5: Life Transitions). They can help the older person to maintain contact with their memories and meaningful life events, and help care staff to see the older person in the context of his or her life, rather than merely as a frail dependent resident.

Once the older person's priorities have been established, the care home should make every effort to facilitate continuity with activities and social contacts. If, for example, the new resident wanted to visit a church, synagogue, or other religious centre once a week, the staff of the home could arrange for someone from the centre to transport the resident. If the older person was too physically frail to undertake a journey, then the priest, rabbi or religious leader should be invited to visit the home at the convenience of the resident. Similar considerations could be given to the person who likes to go out to a public house every Friday evening.

Balancing pre-home lifestyle within a care home setting

The care setting needs to be able to balance the environment to individual differences without making it a home in which older people never know what is going to happen next (Hodgkinson, 1988).

Individuals must be given choices in all aspects of day to day life. This means, for example, that meals could be offered between set times for those who wished to take them. For people who get up late, or like a later supper, there can be means by which they can prepare their own breakfast or supper. Food should not be bland, and choices of ethnic food should always be provided. If a person wants only a slice of bread and butter, or nothing at all, that is what they should have (See Chaper 12: Nutrition).

Sleep patterns also vary between younger and older age. Older people can experience significant changes in their usual sleep patterns following admission to a care home, and a better appreciation of the person's sleep requirements can not only lead to an improvement in well-being, but also a reduction in the amount of sleep medication used (Clapin-French, 1986). Nurses should allow for older people to go to bed when they choose. Televisions, radios or personal headphones can be of great pleasure when the older person cannot get to sleep. Access to tea and other beverages should also be provided during the night hours.

Some older people like to maintain their ability to see to their own financial affairs. Staff should encourage older people to maintain their independence with money (Counsel and Care, 1992). Older people could retain their pension books, collect their own pension, or arrange to have it collected on their behalf.

Staff should also encourage families, friends and visitors, if this is what the older person enjoys. Families can be a good resource and do many things for their older relative. Ebersole and Hess (1990) state that this is especially so if their efforts are perceived as being beneficial and appreciated.

Pets can often expand the sociability of older people and help them to feel needed and loved. Pets also provide tactile comfort, and stroking a dog or cat encourages limb and joint movement. If the continuing care setting cannot keep pets, staff should encourage PAT Dog Schemes. This is a charity that uses volunteer handlers to bring selected dogs into contact with older people.

Satisfaction factors reported by nursing home residents

Various satisfaction factors have been reported by nursing home residents (Ebersole and Hess 1990). These satisfactions included:

● can keep personal possessions,
● something is done about complaints,
● privacy is respected,
● staff show a personal interest,
● nursing staff care about you,
● cheerful place,
● doctor available when needed,
● overall satisfaction,
● help comes within a reasonable time,
● clean room and surroundings,
● good food, and
● choice of bedtime.

These reported satisfactions provide a useful discussion focus for staff within continuing care settings. These satisfactions could be expanded if nursing staff encouraged older people within their settings to add to or prioritise the list.

Individualised care

As early as 1961 Goffman defined characteristics of total institutions. These included:

● all activities in the same place, under the same authority;
● daily activity with a large group of others, all treated the same and required to do the same;
● phases of the day's activities tightly scheduled, imposed rules enforced; and
● all activities designed to meet the aims of the institution.

Detrimental effects of such characteristics will include: sensory deprivation, disorientation, withdrawal, hopelessness, helplessness, loss of identity, deterioration of cognitive functioning and increased dependence.

More recently Stokes and Goudie (1990) suggested that there are many factors in residential care which can be associated with failure to meet individual older people's needs in an environment with little personal contact or stimulation. Such factors include: low morale; lack of enthusiasm; rules and regulations serving the interests of the organisation; lack of information and task-orientated care. Communication is a vital aspect of caring. The ways in which nurses communicate with older people is vitally important because nurses are in a pivotal position in the determination of the quality of people's lives. Despite this, studies have shown that communication between nurses and older people tend to be infrequent and brief, confined to physical care and treatment. (MacLeod-Clark, 1983; Armstrong-Esther, Browne and McAfee, 1994).

Wolfensberger and Thomas (1983) suggest that how a person is perceived and treated by others determines how that person behaves. If a person is seen as passive and unable to make choices and decisions about their care then the less a person expects to have these responsibilities. In contrast to this, the higher the social value accorded to an individual, the greater the expectation for them to make choices.

If nurses spend more time talking to older people, they will learn more about them and their lifestyles. These interactions will do much to enhance opportunities to promote personalised care.

Recreation and leisure

'There is no shortage of things older people in homes can do, and will do, if given the chance', concluded *Counsel and Care's* 1993 survey 'Not only bingo'. The homes in their large sample mentioned 36 different ways of spending time, including arts and crafts, bridge parties and choral singing, theatre visits and walks.

Planning activities for older people living in care homes must obviously strike a balance between:

● the residents' abilities and limitations;
● the variety of residents' desired activities, and the home resources; and
● the skills of current staff, or buying in additional skilled staff for specific activities.

Counsel and Care's survey demonstrated five major objectives when devising a range of home activities:

1. **Combining the maintenance of old interests with the opportunity to explore new ones.** The older people moving into a care home will bring many and diverse skills such as gardening, sewing, cooking or woodcraft. If the home can maximise the sharing of such abilities, residents can enjoy new learning and, at the same time, know they are contributing their expertise to others in the home.
2. **Offering activities which provide physical exercise along with those which encourage mental stimulation.** Recreation and enjoyment can be gained from light-hearted games such as carpet bowls, or from EXTEND exercises (see Chapter 13: Mobility). Older people, even

with disability, can gain immense enjoyment from books (most libraries, or visiting libraries stock large print), from talking books (available on hire from local libraries), or from games which encourage mental agility such as bridge or scrabble.

3. **Providing for individuals as well as groups.** The older people who come into the home may have become accustomed to being with other people, activity, and noise. Alternatively they may be accustomed to solitude and quiet. Residents must have a choice of whether they spend their recreation time alone, or whether they engage with others.

4. **Organisation of regular recurrent activities and one-off events.** There may be residents who have lived alone of necessity but, on moving into a home, find that they want to join with others for specific activities. A regular scheduled programme offers this invitation. One-off events can provide a focus for the residents and staff of the home. Depending on the time of year, many homes offer outings to the seaside or theatre, and plan such events as Summer Fetes or mince pie mornings. These can also encourage local residents, and people of all ages, to maintain the place of the care home within the local community.

5. **Encouraging residents to become involved in organised activity without intruding on individual autonomy.** It could be said that most people have, at some time, wished they had not committed themselves to going somewhere, only to find they had a wonderful time once they had been! If people can experience enjoyment in an activity, they can become more stimulated to participate in future activities. However, some people do not appreciate the idea of activities in the context of old age (Hodgkinson, 1988), and if an individual, despite encouragement, expresses a strong wish **not** to participate, this must be respected and the person supported in his or her decision.

All homes, no matter how small, can offer a variety of recreational and leisure choices. To supplement the participation of some staff in these activities, local volunteers can be a valuable resource. However, because the health needs of individuals will influence the social dimensions of their lives, qualified nurses in the home should always ensure that the resident is not being placed in a situation where he or she is unaware of the risks (see Chapter 6: Rights, Risks and Responsibilites).

An environment that encourages all older people to participate in all activities will produce sensory overload for some, while inactivity can lead to loss of identity, and deterioration in self-esteem, health and will to live.

Older people must be treated as consumers rather than as passive recipients of care. It is important that staff have positive attitudes towards ageing and view ageing as a time when fulfilment and activity are appreciated. Staff need to be committed to provide maximum opportunities for individualised care which include social, leisure and therapeutic opportunities.

Groupwork

Living and working together is all about relationships. In caring for the older person there has been a great change in the nurse–patient relationship from paternalism to partnership. Bringing about this change has taken a long time, and it is still taking place. Small group work is one way of building relationships, based on trust, familiarity and interaction. Groups could be run as either open groups with different residents, or they can be closed groups. Closed groups have the same people in, this encouraging feelings of trust and confidence to share thoughts and feelings. Topics for group work could include fashion, holidays, favourite foods, relaxation, soap operas, wildlife. The range for topics for group-work is very wide (Bender, Norris and Bauckam, 1987; Remocker and Storch, 1987). The nurse's role is to facilitate the group and encourage interaction.

The group will require leadership to explore feelings, reactions and to validate thoughts but this should be sensitive to the individual expressions within the group. Staff members will require training in order to gain confidence when conducting group work. This training is best obtained through participation, discussion and evaluation. The benefits to the daily life in the home will be a greater understanding of each other, a sharing of skills and knowledge between the older people and staff, an improved quality of interactions (Salmon, 1993), and better cohesion within the community. Larger group activities, for instance, fund-raising, charitable giving, national celebrations or theme days will expand into the local community and enhance perceptions of ownership, self-worth and belonging for both the older person and the local community.

Activities and groupwork for people with dementia

People with dementia, even if this is advanced, can participate in social, recreational, leisure, and therapeutic activities. Staff in homes may consider that people with dementia may not be able to participate in these activities because their reality is different to that of the other participants. In fact, people with advanced dementia can participate in, and respond to, environmental opportunities, activities and group work. The challenge is for the nurses to access and understand the reality of the person with dementia, and offer appropriate opportunities. If a sensitive environment is created, individuals with dementia can enjoy many experiences. Examples include walking a path to a seat in the garden.

It is important that nurses attempt to match the kind of activity to the level of ability of the person with dementia. This will enable participants to succeed in being involved. Care must be taken, when simplifying a group activity to suit the abilities of confused older people, not to make the activity childish. When working with older people with dementia, neither under-estimate what they might be able to do, nor place too high an expectation on them. For example, for someone who spends most of their day wandering around the home, getting them to concentrate on an activity for five minutes is a considerable achievement (Bender, Norris and Bauckam, 1987). Small group work for older people with advanced dementia may include food preparation, music, drama, sensory experiences using colour, aromas, sound, touch and taste. Some older people may need a more individual approach to activity. For example, hand massage allows the nurse to touch older people effectively in a very meaningful way. Massage allows the nurse to utilise the skills of touch and comforting associated with caring which can facilitate physical and psychological well-being (Mason, 1988). Some older people enjoy walking, and offering older people the opportunity to wander around a safe environment can help to meet the person's need for activity.

Reminiscence and life review

Many homes organise reminiscence in the belief that older people are happiest when they live in the past. In fact, reminiscence is a normal activity for everybody. Both young and older may choose to reflect on life, or they may not. Coleman (1986) demonstrated that some people enjoyed reminiscing because it enhanced their sense of achievement and meaning of life, others did not because it reinforced their loss of health and independence. A third group chose not to reminisce because they did not want to live in the past.

Reminiscing, whether individually or in a group, can provide opportunities to reflect on life achievements, and can therefore enhance the person's self-esteem and self-worth (Barnat, 1985; Woods, Portnoy, Head and Jones, 1993). It can also provide enjoyment, new learning for those listening to the reminiscences, and a better understanding of the older person's life and experiences.

The participation in reminiscence work must be voluntary and organised by skilled staff who have the knowledge and skills to respond sensitively and appropriately to any emotion evoked by the memories.

Life review may be confused with reminiscence. There are similarities: both reminiscence and life review can occur spontaneously as a response to internally or externally generated thoughts, feelings or sensations. In the context of care homes, life review may be distinguished from reminiscence because it tends to highlight unresolved conflicts, rather than pleasant memories. When these experiences surface, a skilled nurse, who can help the individual to survey and reintegrate the experience, can be beneficial (Hitch, 1994). A helpful analogy can be a drawer which spontaneously springs open. The solution is to take out the clothes, survey, refold and replace them, and close the drawer.

The therapeutic use of activities

In addition to providing recreation and enjoyment, reminiscence can also be used in a therapeutic way by appropriately trained and skilled nurses. Therapeutic reminiscence or life review work may be conducted in an individual way with one nurse and one person towards pre-agreed therapeutic goals (for example working towards the resolution of grief arising from war experiences).

Therapeutic reminiscence groups are carefully planned and structured. They tend to involve the same group of residents, and the same staff in the roles of group facilitator and helper(s). They are usually run at a set time, and at set intervals (for example weekly).

Validation can be used as a therapy or as a communication strategy. The principle is that the nurse respects and validates the feelings being experienced by the older person 'in whatever time or place is real to them at the time, even though it may not correspond to the "here and now" reality' (Bleathman and Morton, 1988).

Residents committees

In principle older people should be encouraged to express their views on the running of the home, and to feel they have as much control as is possible in this. Nurses and home managers will sometimes claim that their residents are too frail to participate in decisions but, in reality, the number of residents who would be unable to express any opinion at all would be a small minority.

Conclusion

This chapter has emphasised that it is possible for nursing staff to create an environment in which older people can spend the last years of their lives in a way which empowers them, and facilitates their choices in as much as can be facilitated within the confines of their individual health and health needs. The chapter has highlighted the opportunities to balance the older person's pre-home lifestyle within the continuing care setting and has emphasised the fundamental importance of positive and creative nursing attitudes in enabling a continuing care environment to empower older people by supporting their independence, their right to freedom of choice and their right to contribute, as fully as possible, in decisions about their lifestyle, environment, activities, and care.

Useful contacts

Age Exchange Reminiscence Centre, 11 Blackheath Village, London SE3 9LA.
Artsline, 5 Crowndale Road, London NW1 1TU.
Council for Music in Hospitals, 74 Queens Road, Hersham, Surrey KT12 5LW.
Disabled Living Foundation, 380–384 Harrow Road, London W9 2HU.
EXTEND (Exercise Training for Elderly and/or Disabled), 1A North Street, Sheringham, Norfolk NR26 8LJ.
Gardens for the Disabled Trust, Hayes Farmhouse, Hayes Lane, Peasmarsh, Rye, East Sussex TN31 6XR.

Holiday Care Service, 2 Old Bank Chambers Station Road, Horley, Surrey RH6 9HW.

Horticultural Therapy, Goulds Ground, Vallis Way, Frome, Somerset BA11 3DW.

Live Music Now, 4 Lower Belgrave Street, London SW1 0LJ.

Magic Me, Mile End Hospital, Bancroft Road, London E1 4DG.

National Listening Library, 12 Lant Street, London SE1 1QH.

National Music and Disability Information Service, Dartington Hall, Totnes, Devon TQ9 6EJ.

The Open College of Arts, Hound Hill, Worsbrough, Barnsley, South Yorkshire S70 6TU.

Talking Book Service, Mount Pleasant, Wembley, Middlesex HA0 1RR.

Talking Newspaper Association (UK), 10 Browning Road, Heathfield, East Sussex TN21 8DB.

University of the Third Age, 1 Stockwell Green, London SW9 9JF.

Winslow Press, Telford Road, Bicester, Oxon OX6 0TS.

The Yoga Biomedical Trust, PO Box 140, Cambridge CB4 3SY.

References

Armstrong-Esther, C.A., Browne, K.D., and McAfee, J.E. (1994) Elderly Patients: Still Clean and Sitting Quietly. *Journal Of Advanced Nursing*, **19**, 264–271.

Barnat, J. (1985) Exploring Living Memory: The Uses of Reminiscence. *Ageing and Society*, **5**, 333–337

Bender, M., Norris, A. and Bauckam, P. (1987) *Groupwork with the Elderly: Principles and Practice*. Bicester, Oxon: Winslow Press.

Bleathman, C. and Morton, I. (1988) Validation Therapy with the Demented Elderly. *Journal of Advanced Nursing*, **13**, 511–514.

Bond J., and Coleman, P. (eds) (1992) *Ageing in Society: An Introduction to Social Gerontology*. London: Sage Publications.

Clapin-French, E. (1986) Sleep Patterns of Aged Persons in Longterm Care Facilities, *Journal of Advanced Nursing*, **11**, 57–66.

Coleman, P.G. (1986) *Ageing and Reminiscence Processes: Social and Clinical Implications*. Chichester: Wiley.

Counsel and Care (1992) *From Home to a Home (A Study of Older People's Hopes, Expectations and Experiences of Residential Care)*. London: Counsel and Care.

Counsel and Care (1993) *Not Only Bingo (A Study of Good Practice in Providing Recreation and Leisure Activities for Older People in Residential Care and Nursing Homes)*. London: Counsel and Care.

Cullinan, T.R. (1991) *Sight*. In S. Redfern (ed.) *Nursing Elderly People*. London: Churchill Livingstone.

Ebersole, P. and Hess, P. (1990) *Towards Healthy Ageing: Human Needs And Nursing Response*. Toronto: C.V. Mosby Co.

Eliopoulos, C. (1993) *Gerontological Nursing*. Philadelphia: J.B. Lippincott Co.

Garland, J. (1991) *Making Residential Care Feel Like Home*. Bicester, Oxon: Winslow Press.

Garrett, G. (1991) Healthy Ageing: Some Nursing Perspectives. London: Wolfe Publishing Ltd.

Goffman, E. (1961) Asylums. New York: Doubleday.

Hitch, S. (1994) Cognitive Therapy as a Tool for Caring for the Elderly Confused Person. *Journal of Clinical Nursing*, **3**, 49–55.

Hodgkinson, J. (1988) *Residential Living: Lifestyle or Life Sentence?* London: Centre For Policy On Ageing.

Johnson, M.L. (1976) That Was Your Life: A Biographical Approach To Later Life. In: V. Carrer and P. Liddiard (eds). *An Ageing Population*. Milton Keynes: Open University Press.

Kane, R.L. et al. (1983) Satisfaction Factors repoeated by Nursing Home Patients. *Journal of Gerontology*, **30**, 385.

MacLeod-Clark (1983) Nurse–patient Communication: An Analysis Of Conversations From Surgical Wards. In: J. Wilson-Barnett (ed.), *Nursing Research. Ten Studies In Patient Care*. Chichester: Wiley.

Mason, A. (1988) Massage. In D. Rankin-Box (ed.) *Complementary Health Therapies: A guide for nurses and the caring professions*. London: Croom Helm.

Redfern, S. (1991) *Nursing Elderly People*. Edinburgh: Churchill Livingstone.

Remocker, A.J. and Storch, E.T. (1987) *Action Speaks Louder: A Handbook of Structured Group Techniques*. London: Churchill Livingstone.

Royal College of Nursing (1993) *Older People And Continuing Care*. London: RCN.

Salmon, P. (1993) Interaction of Nurses with Elderly Patients: Relationship to Nurses' Attitudes and to Formal Activity Periods. *Journal of Advanced Nursing*, **18**, 14–19.

Schofield, I. (1994) Using a Historical Approach to Care. *Elderly Care*, **6**, 6, 14–15.

Schwartz, P.A. (1991) Planning Micro Environments For The Aged. In: E.M. Baines, (ed.). *Perspectives On Gerontological Nursing*. London: Sage Publications.

Sinclair, I. (1988) Residential Care For Elderly People. In: I. Sinclair (ed.) *Residential Care: The Research Reviewed*. (The Wagner Report). London: HMSO

Stokes, G. and Goudie, F. (1990) *Working With Dementia*. Bicester, Oxon: Winslow Press.

Wolfensberger, W. and Thomas, S. (1983) *Program Analysis Of Service Systems Implementation Of Normalisation*. Toronto: Canadian National Institute On Mental Retardation.

Woods, B., Portnoy, S., Head, D. and Jones, G. (1992) Reminiscence and Life Review with Persons with Dementia: Which Way Forward? In: G. Jones and B.M.L. Miesen (eds) *Caregiving in Dementia*. London: Routledge.

Worsley, J. (1992) *Good Care Management: A Guide To Setting Up And Managing A Residential Home*. ACE Books. Age Concern, England.

Yurick, A.G., Spier, B.E., Robb, S.S. and Ebert, N.J. (1989) *The Aged Person and The Nursing Process*. California: Appleton and Lange.

Further Reading

Armstrong, J. (1987) *Staying Active: A Positive Approach In Residential Homes*. Centre For Policy On Ageing. Dorset: Dorset Press.

Baines, E.M. (1991) *Perspectives On Gerontological Nursing*. London: Sage Publications.

Burnside, I.M. (1988) *Nursing and The Aged: A Self Care Approach*. London: McGraw-Hill Book Co.

Garland, J. (1991) *Making Residential Care Feel Like Home*. Bicester, Oxon: Winslow Press.

Gearing, B. and Dant, T. (1990) Doing Biographical Research. In: S.M. Peace. (ed.) *Researching Social Gerontology*. London: Sage.

Hodgkinson, J. (1988) *The Admission Process*. London: Centre For Policy on Ageing.

Hodgkinson, J. (1988) *Encouraging Residents' Activities*. London: Centre For Policy on Ageing.

Hogstel, M. (1990) *Geropsychiatric Nursing*. Toronto: C.V. Mosby Co.

Jones, G. and Miesen B.M.L. (1992) *Care Giving in Dementia: Research and Applications*. London: Routledge.

Netten, A. (1993) *A Positive Environment? Physical and Social Influences On People With Senile Dementia In Residential Care*. Cambridge: Cambridge University Press.

Norris, A. (1986) *Reminiscence*. London: Winslow Press.

Sinclair, I. (1988) *Residential Care: The Research Reviewed* (The Wagner Report). London: HMSO.

8

Management Matters

Steve Goodwin

Introduction

Nurses joining the management team of a nursing home are likely to be called upon to manage situations and take responsibility for issues that they have seldom met before. Even where nurses have previously held senior positions and had high levels of responsibility elsewhere, they may still be surprised at the broad base of management and administration duties in a care home setting. They will require an all embracing approach that will often test their experience and inter-personal skills.

The registering authority for the home will have requirements regarding the staffing of the home. Currently these requirements are governed by health authority registration and inspection for nursing homes and local authority registration and inspection for residential homes. If a home has dual registration then both registration and inspection units will be involved. (see Chapter 1). Nurses who work in residential care homes have long argued that they should be free to practice as nurses. The UKCC (1992a) refers to nurses working in this sector in its Scope of Professional Practice, paragraphs 20 and 21. It specifically refers to nurses who are employed in posts which do not require nursing qualifications. This will often mean that quite junior nurses may be required to manage and take responsibility for the home for part or the whole of a shift. Nurses who have previously been employed in hospital settings, or who have only worked in very small teams, are not likely to have experienced the management of a broad-based, multi-skilled team of the type frequently found in larger care homes. These teams may include differing grades of nursing and care staff, administrative and clerical staff, housekeeping and laundry teams, qualified chefs and other catering or kitchen staff. Also to be found in many homes are gardeners, maintenance and handy-persons all of whom have key roles in keeping complex plant and building fabric in safe and working order. It is important to reflect upon this broad band of respon-sibility because even nurses working for as little as one night a week may soon find that it is on their particular shift that the lift decides to fail, or the washing machine floods. They may be called to handle a complaint about supper, or deal with an unannounced inspection team visit in the middle of the night.

Working within a domestic environment

Before discussing some of the varied management issues that may arise for nurses occupying various roles in care homes, it is important to emphasise that nurses will be working in an environment which is home to its residents. Residents' needs will not always be primarily clinical, but will revolve much more around their living environment, activities of daily living and quality of life. All this will be fashioned from moment to moment on the emotional anvil of institutional living. It is also worth considering that most of the people who live within the home will also die there. These people are likely to have given up a home in recent times as well as around 95 per cent of their possessions. Add to this that many will be funding themselves thus becoming the nurses' employers, albeit indirectly. Residents have their own expectations to which the whole home team will need to respond. Nurses will also be governed by their professional body (see Chapter 3), the requirements of the home owner and the wider statutory implications enforced by the registering authority. Nurses trying to adhere to all these persuasions can often struggle to find a management style and approach that reflects the domestic setting in which they operate, yet complies with the clinical, legislative and professional responsibilities that their presence dictates.

Planning for effective management

The key approaches in managing any span of duty in a care home requires much more thought and vision than is required just to get through without anything going wrong, however much of a blessing this may seem at the end of a busy day or night. Good management within a home will have a commitment and a purpose. There will be strategies for when things go wrong, and practice guidelines to put things right. Team decisions will create short- and long-term plans to take care practices forward. Nurses must also operate in such a manner that all the co-ordination, planning and implementation that these considerations demand is not obtrusive to the people who live there. The management and administration of a home requires calm control and quiet efficiency. A home that is constantly being held together by panic measures, where nurses and carers work at a constant fast pace just to survive, may appear a stimulating and thriving place to work. To live there may be at times quite unbearable. As one might expect, most care homes are very busy places to work. Homes that constantly function on red alert may need management investigation, as well as regular evaluation of work practices and overall organisation. Although the pendulum of management may continue, if nurses derive little pleasure from their busy activities, then the pleasant chimes of success will rarely be heard as time rushes by. On some days, getting through and getting by is the best that can be hoped for, but this no strategy for developing practices that will achieve a better quality of life for those who live there.

Planning around the needs of residents

Many of the key management issues in a home surround the management of people whether they live, work or visit there. Giving consideration to the priorities, needs and expectations of these parties is important.
These can often differ and even collide. The greater the amounts of
choice, autonomy and control placed with residents, the more this will
affect the way in which all members of the home team operate. Families
and visitors may have their own views on how things should operate,
and the interface between these different groups can often lead to
tensions, or even conflicts. A home that is resident focused will be flexible
in its organisation and approach to residents' care. It will arrange the
routines and activities in direct response to the changing needs of individual residents, wherever opportunities to do so arise.

Residents' care plans: prioritising needs

Residents' individual care plans must reflect how each person's care will
be managed on a day to day basis. This will then direct and define how
staff (and to a certain extent, families) will behave and operate around
that person. It will influence care practices, correct approaches, and the
level and amount of contact each grade of staff may need to have.
Relatives and significant others may also have a key part to play, and the
care plan must be compiled accordingly. The aims and intentions of both
staff and families can be brought together in the care plan in simple terms
of what needs to be done to assist the resident to arrive at the goals they
themselves have set. In this way relatives and friends can participate,
comment and be helped to understand why certain aspects of care are
carried out in particular ways. A relative may otherwise, for example, not
grasp why mother was encouraged to dress herself or is taken to the
dining room in a wheel chair. What to a nurse may be good practices of
rehabilitation may, to a visitor, appear to be the result of staff shortages
or even a lack of care. The expectation of many families is that their
relative is to have things done for them or why would they be paying
such a fee? Many complaints and grievances grow from these basic but
important differing perceptions of need and expectations.

   The care plan is a vital and useful nursing tool in prioritising and planning care. It is the essential guide as to how the home will need to be
organised, and what resources will be needed on a day to day basis. The
care plan will also need to reflect that which can reasonably be achieved
with the resources made available. It is not constructive to aim to reach
goals that will require intensive nursing input that cannot consistently be
guaranteed. Nurses as managers may reach a stage from time to time
where they need to be particularly careful that the dependency and level
of care required by newly admitted and existing residents do not outstrip
their resources. The nursing team will need to operate with decisiveness
and accurate criteria when this stage is reached, and some sick or frail
people may have to be deemed unsuitable for admission while those
circumstances prevail. Turning down prospective clients is rarely a

popular decision for any of the parties concerned, especially so in times where the home's high occupancy is an economic necessity or alternatively where an immediate transfer from hospital to release a bed is vital. Nurses who manage this (often precarious) balancing act will also have to contend with the statutory requirements laid down by the registering authority, and the often prescriptive budgets set by their employers.

Managing the staff resource

Defining the staff working roster as a created thing may seem odd as, in most establishments, with frequent changes, it is often better perceived as something that is continuously evolving. Some nurses revert to the system they last used in hospital. Progressively, in a bid to keep everyone satisfied, the record becomes less and less recognisable with all the frantic pencilling in and rubbing out. By the end of the week managers are left trying to decipher who was where and when. Firstly, the staffing roster is not to be considered as the 'off-duty'. It is a record and plan of how staff resources are to be best utilised to meet care needs, and to maintain the safety and comfort of the people who live there and who indirectly employ the staff. It should primarily establish when staff are required, not how to achieve their time off. Of course, trying to build in some flexibility to help staff with their wider family and social commitments may be achievable, and a certain degree of give and take is crucial.

Setting up the duty roster is a priority task that will take time. Staff of all grades are the home's most important resource. They accommodate around 45 per cent of the entire budget, and it is prudent to make best use of their time and endeavours. It is always difficult to make changes to existing and long-standing duty arrangements but it is well worth striving to make changes that reap benefits to residents' care. Setting off in the right direction can be achieved at the selection interview by being clear about what commitment and flexibility is required. There will also need to be a good mix of part and full time staff, as well as a reliable bank of competent casual staff. Many management and disciplinary issues that arise in a home stem from the fact that there has been little scope and thought given to the selection, planning and deployment of staff. The registering authority will also wish to view the staffing rota, and may even request that a copy is sent to them monthly. This will help indicate to them how the home has complied with the statutory requirements, and will also indicate how the staff resource is being managed and organised.

The numbers and grades of staff required on duty throughout a 24-hour period will often be quite prescriptively set out by the registering authority. A copy of this should be at hand to refer to. Failure to comply can lead to further action being taken and even possible prosecution under the 1984 Registered Homes Act. Many authorities clearly indicate the number of first- and second-level nurses as well as care staff. Other grades of staff are also required and the authority's inspection team may want clarity on how tasks and responsibilities differ between care staff, and domestic or laundry teams. This is especially the case in smaller homes where there is often a greater cross-over of roles and duties. All grades of staff, particularly managers, need to be rostered for when they will be of best service to the residents and the home in general. For a manager and administrator this may well be at weekends or evenings. Many domestic and housekeeping duties are best carried out during the evening or night especially the cleaning of lounges, dining areas and kitchens.

Depending on where the machines are located, the laundry may also operate at night. Toilets should be clean and ready for use at all times. The views of residents and visitors will help decide how and when staff are best deployed and these issues should be regularly discussed at staff meetings.

Finding the right people

When staff vacancies occur, then full consideration can be given to creating new posts and modified ways of working that more closely reflect the residents' changing needs, wishes and suggestions. When appointing staff to the home, nurses should make sure appointments are well thought out and that the selection process is consistent and fair so that suitable staff are appointed. Consideration also needs to be given to the balance and mix of staff in terms of experience, and numbers of younger or more mature staff. Sadly, too little time is often invested in the selection and recruitment of care and housekeeping staff. Interviews should be well planned and test the true knowledge, experience and attitude of all the candidates fairly and openly. Applicants should have a job profile before the interview, and those on the selection panel should be clear about who and what they are looking for. Many home managers and other nurses spend more time choosing the fixtures and fittings for the home than they do in selecting the staff. They subsequently waste valuable time trying to rectify staffing problems and care practices that have stemmed from making the wrong appointment. When staff are appointed there must be an induction programme for them (UKCC, 1994). Not only is this fair and proper for them, the people they will be caring for and their work colleagues, but it can avoid safety and management problems if they are properly inducted.

Induction packs can be easily put together and improved upon by feedback from new staff, or alternatively they may be bought as part of specially designed packages for nursing home use.

Developing individual staff and building teams

Nurses in charge of a home, even for a shift, have the responsibility, not only for themselves, but also for those around them and especially for those under their direct supervision. Make sure staff have a clear understanding of their role, and the responsibility within that role. This will require that every staff member has a job outline, even if they have been working at the home for some time without one. Discuss roles and work practices regularly at staff meetings. Explore views and perceptions of how roles are closely related between the different disciplines in the home. This is not just the case with care and housekeeping staff, but particularly so between nursing and care staff. For a large part of the day, care staff and qualified nursing staff carry out very largely similar duties and activities. There needs to be clear understanding of why this is and how levels of accountability differ. It is also important to explore why duties that appear similar may have different values placed upon them when carried out by a trained or qualified practitioner.

It is unlikely that pay will ever really reflect the true value placed on good care staff. Regular encouragement, and seeking opportunities to make their roles and duties more interesting is necessary. Sharing learning opportunities and developing practice and research findings if explained appropriately is of much value and interest to many of them. Care staff are a wealth of information and ideas and may be better acquainted with quality of life issues of residents than many nursing staff.

Planning a 24-hour approach to care

Routines and rituals and care

Managing the night period requires no less capability than that of any other period. Rotation of staff between various shifts will help many get an enlightened view of what the priorities of care are across the day and night periods. This can also highlight how differently the needs or behaviours of some residents change as the day progresses. There are often different levels of interaction between staff and residents during the latter part of the day, and the night. The routine of the home strongly influences the lifestyle and quality of life of most residents. Their care is affected by levels of staff and shift patterns. Drug administration, mealtimes, bed-times, drinks and the times residents are awakened or assisted to get up: indeed, many aspects of the day to day lifestyles of residents have to correspond with staff activity and availability. The challenge is to develop a healthy balance between the needs of the residents and the need for routine within a care home. Consideration of the ease with which ritualised care can develop, care which only meets the needs of the staff, will promote healthy discussion and questioning of care practices (Walsh and Ford, 1989; Ford and Walsh, 1994).

Care planning is as important during the night as it is during the day period. Reports should give an accurate account about what has happened during the night. Many older people living in care homes do suffer from sleep disruptions and other care issues that affect their quality of life such as pain, cramps, confusion, and often fearfulness or loneliness. The night care team can bring about improvements which will benefit residents in diverse ways simply by investigating the suitability of beds, linen and pillows, noise levels, room temperatures, light interference, and the effects of boredom or even hunger. The list seems almost endless, which is why having nothing significant to report seems some-what odd night after night.

Competent and confident staff

Update of clinical skills for night nurses is particularly important. They are often called upon to make key clinical and diagnostic decisions that will affect the necessity to call out a doctor, or to request the assistance of the emergency services. On many occasions there may only be one quali-fied nurse on duty at night. It is at times like this that the nurse may really miss the support and advice often at hand for their colleagues in hospital or larger homes. The decision to call out a GP at night may, for some nurses, be done with little hesitation, while others may agonise before reaching a decision. Although this may, to some, seem a quite straight-forward decision clinically, it does also carry some management implica-tions in terms of how they handle an awkward or reluctant doctor. Once a decision has been clinically arrived at by the nurse, and as is often the case with nursing older people this is in itself a highly skilled task, then the necessary medical assistance should be summoned. Nurses need not be apologetic about seeking medical help at any time of day or night. Keeping a clear record of the circumstances and situation that has led up to the decision being made will help the nurse to convince the doctor that their presence is required. It may also be of some benefit at a future date when a colleague finds themselves in a similar situation. A clear, concise and accurate record of events can't guarantee that a nurse will always make the right decision, but it may well avoid them and the doctor making the wrong one, especially if the doctor is half awake at the other end of the phone.

Support of other agencies

The care home team will require from time to time the input of various agencies and health professionals. Many of these will be nurses with specialist roles, and particular knowledge and clinical expertise. These will include the community psychiatric nurse, tissue viability nurse, continence adviser and infection control nurses. The availability, location and referral method for these and other agencies will vary from region to region. Services such as physiotherapy, occupational and speech therapy, and to a certain extent chiropody, can be more difficult to arrange in some areas unless private funds can be made available to buy them in. The NHSE (1995) guidelines on health authorities' responsibilites should facilitate the access to, and funding of, such services. Dentists and opti-cians will carry out domiciliary visits to the home though some may charge or only offer a limited service. In all cases, perseverance to find the best and most willing service usually pays dividends.

As an increasing number of residents are being referred by the local authority, then the involvement of social workers and their counterparts the care managers and locality managers will be more apparent. Many of these people will have a good rapport with the resident and prove to be a valuable resource for information and advice.

The role that the general practitioner adopts will also have its effect on the overall health and well-being of residents. Finding the right working relationship between the GP practice and the homes' nursing team is not always easy. Some doctors will be pleased to call any day whilst others prefer to hold weekly clinics in the home or only come at the direct request of the nursing team. Residents will have their own expectations of what they require of their doctor; some will not know their GP well because they may have had to change practices as part of their admission. There is always some benefit from nurses sitting down with the doctor and their patient to discuss plans of care and the priorities that stem from it. From this an outline of what roles the differing professionals and other staff will play can be agreed upon. It is important that the resident and their family is involved and informed in respect of this, even where the patient has communication difficulties or dementia.

On occasions, help and advice from professional bodies such as the Royal College of Nursing or the Registered Nursing Homes Association may prove invaluable. Along with other local and national interest groups they house a wealth of expertise, research findings and provide useful networks and information packs (RCN 1996a,b). The registration and inspection teams are also often willing to give practical advice and support, and are keen not just to be seen in the mode of compliance and policing the statutory requirements.

Statutory requirements

Most nurses working in care homes will know that the home has to be registered with the local health authority as directed under the Registered Homes Act, 1984, in England and Wales and its equivilent in Northern Ireland and Scotland (see Chapter 1). The authority are required to visit the home for inspection purposes and most do so at least twice annually. One visit is usually pre-arranged with the home whilst the other is made unannounced. The inspection team has the right of entry at any time and can request to see documentation relevant to their sphere of responsibility. They will also follow up complaints made to them and will almost certainly need to view nursing reports, care plans, staffing rotas, and records pertaining to fire, health and safety, accidents and other reportable incidents. Nursing and pharmacy staff attached to the inspection team may also carry out checks to the drug and medicines administration systems and records, and some guidance regarding standards for administration has been issued (UKCC, 1992b) (see Chapter 16). A copy of the inspection team's documentation for standards and requirements under the Acts can help nurses better understand the broad base of their own responsibilities and most teams would be pleased to give a copy of this to any nurse who so requests. Nurses should also familiarise themselves with previous inspection reports as there may be issues they wish to have qualified or wish to respond to.

Part of the inspection visit may focus upon how residents' affairs are managed. There are times when nurses need to handle residents' fees and monies, or their pensions. Clear directives for financial procedures need to be operational if this is the case. Records of residents' own finances, fees and contracts of residence should be kept separate from other nursing and care reports. These should not be made available to nursing staff unless the resident has directed the home manager to do so. A nurse may be encouraged to show prospective residents or their families around the home, but details of fees and contracts should really be discussed with the manager or administrator.

Health and safety issues

An important part of being in charge of a nursing home is to create a safe, comfortable and stimulating environment. Here clinical practice will be carried out in what is primarily a domestic and homely setting. A knowledge of the key issues surrounding health and safety is essential. The home must have clear policies in operation for issues such as fire, lifting and handling of residents, food hygiene and the usage and storage of potentially hazardous materials including clinical waste. These policies must be constantly monitored and all grades of staff must be updated and trained in respect of changes in law and working practices. Particular thought and planning needs to be given where frail elderly, disabled and confused people live. Do not allow opinion to dictate that which can be decided as a matter of fact. Always record and highlight any issue that remains unresolved between agencies or individuals. Nurses should also make use of guidance on standards for record keeping (UKCC, 1993).

Often Fire Officers require standards of safety practice that can create care problems for residents and staff, particularly issues concerning fire doors and evacuation requirements. Keep discussions going until satisfactory arrangements are reached, ensuring residents' viewpoints are not excluded. Consideration may also have to be given to pets in a home. Their management and welfare is important too; check that they are being well cared for and not creating a risk or nuisance to others. Pets can create hazards but, if properly managed and cared for, they can prove to be valuable members of the team. They often are less discriminative and more forgiving than many of the professionals when it comes to the care of older people.

Staff themselves often create hazardous situations just by the inadequacy of what they wear. Ensure therefore that suitable footwear is worn at all times and that uniforms or suitable alternatives provide adequate protection and are not uncomfortable to wear or be seen in. There is a need for special care and planning when building and repair work is taking place in a home or its grounds. Extra diligence will need to be paid and particular focus given to residents who have sensory impairments or are confused (see Chapter 7). There are added dimensions to working nights in a care home that will not be familiar to those who have worked largely in hospitals or on the community. These are the issues surrounding security. A home that is located in a rural locality may be no more vulnerable to intruders or crime than that in a built up area, but it can certainly make staff feel that is the case. The night nurse in charge will carry a large responsibility for the safety of residents and staff. They should always have at hand contacts for police and other useful help. Doors and windows should be fitted with locks, and curtains must be able to be drawn. Car parks and staff passages should have adequate lighting, and staff who need to venture out during periods of darkness should not go unaccompanied.

Crime prevention officers from the local police will gladly advise on safe working practices in care homes and add weight when there seems a reluctance for owners or managers to make improvements in this area. Prompt reporting in writing is important when lights and locks are broken or inadequate. Nursing homes should adopt a security policy that is monitored and updated regularly. There are many unexpected incidents that can occur during the night within nursing homes. Those who take charge need to be prepared for things to suddenly, and even drastically, go wrong from time to time. It is therefore important to develop and have at hand policies and practice guidelines that will help if and when these occur.

Particularly helpful will be operational directives for when a lift fails, calling out a GP at night, or requesting the emergency services, sudden death of a resident, emergency admission to the home or transfer to hospital. Simple directives save time. For example can escort staff get a taxi back if a resident is admitted through accident and emergency? If so where will they get the fare from? What may be of no great issue on the day shift could still be of great significance on nights where an absent staff member can mean a real disruption, and even put some element of risk to the remainder of the home. It sounds obvious to state that nurses should not wait for things to go wrong, but all too often they are left scrambling around for contact numbers, or wading through great thick files to locate the appropriate information.

Conclusion: finding out how you manage

Nurses who seek to have their management and clinical skills developed will find the home environment a real testing ground. Here they will have to learn to adopt, and to foster a style and approach that reflects the sensitive nature of their work. They will work in a largely domestic setting that is first and foremost the place that many people call home. Amidst the hurly-burly of day to day activity they will be required to bring and establish a calm control. This should help distract from the immense activity that is generated from the often frantic interface of all those who live, work or visit there. Little of the chemistry of all this takes place in some hidden management laboratory such as an office or nurses' station. The cut and thrust of care management brings most nurses into close and direct contact with the very people who are the focus of their attention and responsibility.

References

DHSS (1984) Registered Homes Act 1984. London: HMSO.

Ford, P. and Walsh, M. (1994) *New rituals for old, nursing through the looking glass*. Oxford: Butterworth-Heinemann.

NHS Executive (1995) Responsibilities for meeting long term care needs. HSG(94).

Royal College of Nursing (1996a) *Nursing Skills: Nursing Values*. London: RCN Publishing.

Royal College of Nursing (1996b) *Good Employment Practice in Nursing Homes*. London: RCN Publishing.

United Kingdom Central Council (1992a) The Scope of Professional Practice. UKCC.

United Kingdom Central Council (1992b) Standards for the administration of medicines. UKCC.

United Kingdom Central Council (1993) Standards for records and record keeping. UKCC.

United Kingdom Central Council (1994) Professional Conduct – Occasional Report on Standards of Nursing in Nursing homes. UKCC.

Walsh, M. and Ford, P. (1989) *Nursing Rituals, Research and Rational Actions*. Oxford: Butterworth-Heinemann.

Further reading

Cartwright, Collins, Green and Candy (1993) *Managing Finance and Information*. Oxford: Blackwells.

Collins, H. (1993) *Human Resources Management*. London: Hodder and Stoughton.

Cook, S. (1993) *Customer Care*. London: Kogan Page.

Crawley, R. (1994) *Performance Appraisal*. London: Lemos Associates.

Drucker, P. (1993) *Managing in Turbulent Times*. Oxford: Butterworth-Heinemann.

Fowler, A. (1990) *A Good Start (Effective Employee Induction)*. Exeter: Short Run Press.

Hague, P. (1993) *Interviewing*. London: Kogan Page.

Karlof, B. (1993) *Key Business Concepts*. London: Routledge Publications.

Lucey, T. (1994) *Business Administration*. London: D.P. Publications.

Malone, M. (1992) *Your Employment Rights*. London: Kogan Page.

Moon, P. (1993) *Appraising Your Staff*. London: Kogan Page.

Parry, H. (1991) *Meetings*. London: Croner Publications.

Pheasant, S. (1991) *Ergonomics, Work and Health*. London: Macmillan.

Rae, L. (1990) *The Skills of Interviewing*. Aldershot: Gower.

Sheal, P.R. (1994) *How to Develop and Present Staff Training Courses*. London: Kogan Page.

Stranks, J. (1992) *A Manager's Guide to Health and Safety at Work*. London: Kogan Page.

Walker, D. (1994) *Customer First*. Aldershot: Gower.

Wauld, C. (1991) *Daily Mail Employment Law*. London: Chapmans Publishers.

9

Educational Issues

Irene Schofield

Introduction

Education in care homes has two dimensions. The first is that of education for the staff who are employed to deliver care. It is generally agreed that education and training can play a key role in changing the attitudes and work practices of professional carers and 'give vision to the purpose and potential of later life' (Phillipson and Strang, 1986). The second dimension is that of education for the residents themselves. This encompasses health education in terms of maintaining well-being in the presence of chronic illness and disability, and the prevention of complications. It also includes the need to be mentally and physically active and creative, within the confines of disability. No care can be considered to be of a high standard unless the requirement for creativity and individual continuing development is met.

Education and training for staff

It is appropriate to open this chapter with some salutary words from Doreen Norton, a pioneer in the development of the care of older people as a specialist nursing activity. She suggested that the care of older people had been 'one of ignorance and educational neglect' by the nursing profession itself, and that it was commonly described as 'only basic nursing', requiring little knowledge or skill on the part of the care giver. Furthermore, she questioned the common premise that, because the majority of patients and clients were older people, then this was sufficient in itself to prepare nurses to care for their special needs (Norton, 1990).

However, the age of enlightenment is slowly beginning to dawn with the growing recognition that older people have complex needs as a result of biological age-related changes, multiple pathology, and psychosocial changes specific to the later stages of the life-span continuum. Therefore, it is essential that nurses must be equipped with the appropriate knowledge and skills to be able to deliver quality care to older people.

A recent report (DoH, 1994) describes education and training for nurses as 'the bedrock of professional practice which aims to provide the highest standards of care'. The report is primarily concerned with nurses working in the health service but these words are equally applicable to nurses working in care homes, or other facilities which exist to provide continuing care for older people. In addition, some recent changes in nurse education will facilitate this process of preparation.

Wherever they work, professional nurses are subject to the rules relating to competence to practice. The Code of Professional Conduct (UKCC, 1992a) states that nurses have a duty to maintain and improve their professional competence and knowledge. From 1995 this is mandatory so that, in order to remain on the register, nurses will have to undertake a specific period of continuing development in order to update their skills. In addition, The Scope of Professional Practice (UKCC, 1992b) acknowledges the dynamic nature of health-care requirements, and lays down guiding principles for nurses taking on new roles. The document also reminds practitioners that these principles apply to nurses working in personal social services or residential homes, who elect to carry out care delegated, for example, by community nurses.

Nurses who work in situations of relative professional isolation may face particular challenges. A report by the nurses' professional body (UKCC, 1994b) gives examples of misconduct by professional nurses working in nursing homes. It recommends that all grades of staff should receive an induction programme immediately on starting employment, have regular in-service training, and access to relevant external courses. It also recommended that newly-qualified staff are supported, and that those nurses returning to practice after a specified break should be updated as regards current issues. Care homes will increasingly become the main source of continuing support for those older people who are too frail to remain in their own homes. It is vital that this care is provided by teams lead by skilled nurses whose care is research-based and who can create a working environment which is conducive and supportive to all grades of staff.

Current developments in continuing education

Current thinking about nurse education acknowledges that pre-registration education is truly just the beginning, and that the dynamic nature of health-care requires nurses to subscribe to the idea of life-long learning. From April 1995, PREP (Post Registration Education and Practice) came into being as the formal framework for continuing education. In addition, there are other more informal methods by which nurses can take responsibility for their own learning.

PREP

There are three major sets of requirements. These are preceptorship, professional competence, and specialist or advanced practice.

Preceptorship

Firstly, there is a recommended period of four months, during which a newly qualified nurse should work under the guidance of a preceptor before taking on the full responsibilities of the new role. This has implications for homes where there may only be one registered nurse on duty at a time. A learning contract linked to requirements of the newly qualified nurse's job description and formulated as a result of discussion between nurse and preceptor could be a way around this. Also, if the nurse is to take charge of the home within the period of preceptorship, the contact number of the preceptor or another experienced qualified member of staff could be provided as backup. It should be made clear that it is acceptable to ask for help.

Many nurses will not have had the opportunity to work in care homes during their initial period of training. Unlike hospital settings, where there are senior colleagues and peers at hand from whom to seek advice, new nurses are in charge on their own. It is important that this is recognised by employees and matrons, so that systems are devised to provide support, albeit from a distance.

Professional competence

The second requirement is statutory and states that all registered nurses (first and second level) must provide evidence of maintaining and developing professional knowledge and competence. In practical terms this means that applications to remain on the UKCC register, must be supported by evidence of attending a minimum of five study days every three years, employment information, and a personal professional profile. In the future, nurses who have had a break from practice for five years or more will be required to have completed a Return to Practice programme. A period of supervised practice will be an integral part of such schemes, and hospitals and care homes may be asked to provide it. The laws of supply and demand for qualified nurses may affect who funds such programmes – the individual nurse or the prospective employer.

The UKCC has established five categories of study for the achievement of PREP requirements of five study days over the three year period of registration. Topics chosen should relate to the care of patients within the nurse's area of employment. The categories are as follows:

1. **Reducing risk:** relates to the identification of health problems, the protection of individuals at risk of ill health, and risk reduction by health promotion and screening. Topics relevant to home care might be an update on infection control, how to manage an outbreak of diarrhoea, accident prevention, gentle exercise for frail older adults, healthy eating and strategies to help people adjust to living in communal surroundings.
2. **Care enhancement:** incorporates developments in clinical practice and treatment, such as continence promotion and management, and pressure sore prevention. Standard setting is already being carried out by group-owned homes but small homes may also wish to embark on setting their own standards. Empowering consumers could involve a session on consideration of rights and risks in the care of frail older people or setting up and facilitating a residents' committee.

3. **Patient, client and colleague support:** encompasses counselling and leadership skills. These are essential to effective communication with any client group, but there are particular challenges in relating to people with impaired hearing and sight, and mental impairments. Specialist therapeutic approaches such as facilitation of life review, reminiscence and validation, and support for the bereaved and dying could be considered in this category. Sessions on leadership skills contribute to the retention, satisfaction and happiness of staff, whilst guidance on stress management, for both staff and residents, are important to those working and living in relatively closed environments, often without immediate peer support.

4. **Practice development:** includes external visits which might be to another home to see how care is delivered in a different environment, to a hospice, or to a provider of equipment such as the Disabled Living Foundation, with a view to evaluating new equipment. Time can be devoted to personal research or study, prior to initiating a practice change. Briefing on health and policy change and service audit is also considered appropriate. Such briefing meetings may be of short duration but nevertheless should be recorded in the nurse's personal and professional development profile. The date, length of time taken and session should all be documented followed by a short account of what has been covered and its implications for nursing practice.

5. **Educational development:** covers teaching and learning skills, both for the benefit of staff and residents or clients. The ENB 998 Course Teaching and Assessing in Clinical Practice, and City and Guilds 730 Further Education Teacher's Certificate are recognised qualifications. Sessions on running groups for older people are sometimes offered by local authority health promotion departments, and material on teaching and learning for older adults is mainly offered as part of a longer course.

These are just a few suggestions as to how the PREP requirements for periodic registration might be met; the list is not exhaustive. Neither is it intended that development necessarily involves whole days away from the workplace. The important thing is that sessions are accurately documented and validated.

The personal professional profile   The use of a professional profile or portfolio is also a mandatory requirement by the UKCC. Nurses will be required to keep written records to demonstrate their continuing development of professional knowledge and competence. The profile will comprise key personal and professional details, including pre- and post-registration education, employment history, responsibilities and opportunities in posts held, and how these contribute to professional development and improved client care. There will be space for analysis of critical incidents and reflection on current practice, as well as action plans for the acquisition of new skills and competencies. There are already pro-forma portfolios available for purchase from, for example, the Welsh National Board, the Royal College of Nursing or nursing journals, but nurses can also construct their own, so long as the UKCC requirements are met.

Paying for PREP   Lastly, it is important to consider who is responsible for ensuring that the PREP requirements are met. The UKCC states clearly that it is the responsibility of each individual nurse to ensure that the requirements are met, although they also say they hope that employers will support staff in respect of giving time and/or financial support. Eaves (1988) puts forward an excellent framework for establishing the educational needs of all grades of staff, and also suggests that everyone is responsible for continuing education, including the proprietor, nurse, and inspection bodies. Proprietors need to acknowledge that education and training are routes to quality care, and that they are worth the investment. It is vital that care home residents are nursed by appropriately-trained staff, and such a requirement should be included in local authority purchasing contract specifications.

The following topics are suggested as a basis for an education programme for qualified nurses in care homes:

- normal ageing,
- manual handling update,
- entering a nursing home/managing the transition,
- update on approaches to caring for people with dementia,
- managing challenging behaviours,
- continence care/management of incontinence,
- facilitating choice/managing rights and risks,
- common medications and their effects on older people,
- teamwork and leadership skills,
- models of care appropriate to nursing homes/supported housing,
- stress management,
- terminal care to include advances in pain control
- health education in continuing care, and
- diabetes update.

Specialist and advanced practice

The third and final requirement relates to standards for the preparation of the **specialist practitioner**, successful achievement of which will be recorded on the UKCC register. It is recommended that programmes will be one academic year in length, be no less than first degree level and offer credit for prior experiential learning (APEL or APL), be modular and flexible and accessible on a full- or part-time basis. The programme should have clearly defined outcomes and be approved by a National Board. Examples would be the BSc in Nursing Studies incorporating the English National Board Higher Award, or the Scottish National Board qualification in Professional Studies. It is appropriate for the matron or nurse in charge to be registered as a specialist practitioner in the care of the older adult.

The PREP document also discusses **advanced practice**, whereby nurses are prepared at a level to enable them to advance practice in terms of research, management and education, and to contribute to the formulation of policy. The document suggests that academic study at masters degree level would be suitable preparation. Increasingly masters degrees, often of a multidisciplinary nature and relating to the care of older people, are being offered around the country. Nurses holding senior positions in care home groups should ideally be prepared at this level.

The use of reflection in nursing practice and management

Reflection is now incorporated as a method of learning in many pre- and post-registration courses. However, for nurses who qualified some time ago the concept is unfamiliar. It is a process which is based on the exploration and evaluation of specific incidents and situations arising from everyday practice. Reflection is an equally valuable tool for nursing home managers as it is for practitioners. Reflection also provides a framework for personal and professional development of the nurse, as well as for review of nursing and management practice within the home. Reflection also facilitates the setting and evaluation of individual objectives which can form the basis for IPR (Individual Performance Review).

Clinical supervision

Clinical supervision is a means of enabling nurses to develop their professional practice for the benefit of residents and clients in their care. It is a formal process, whereby the nurse meets regularly with an experienced colleague, to discuss and reflect on chosen aspects of her/his work. Integral to clinical supervision is a trusting and respectful relationship with the supervisor, and a willingness to develop skills in assessment, analysis and reflection (NHS Management Executive, 1993).

Clinical supervision may be difficult to achieve in small nursing homes, where there is usually only one qualified nurse on duty. One way forward could be to develop a network of professional support with nurses in other homes. An important consideration when forging links between homes is the risk of passing on commercially sensitive information. This could be dealt with by establishing preliminary ground rules, which prohibit the discussion of certain types of information.

Creating a learning environment

An important aspect of the qualified nurse's role is the supervision and continuing education and training of the unqualified care staff. Any opportunity should be taken to expand their knowledge and skills, and to encourage a questioning approach to their work. This can be done while working alongside residents, if appropriate, or at handover times. A notice board for educational articles of relevance to the care of specific residents could be maintained by qualified staff.

Guidelines for good practice

Managers/proprietors

● Make an action plan for education and training as part of your annual plan.

Nurses

● Develop the habit of life-long learning. It's never too late.
● Get into the habit of setting time aside each month to read a journal article relevant to your work.
● Discuss with your manager how you might put new ideas into practice.

Health care support workers/nursing assistants/care assistants

Registered nurses usually form only a small part of the workforce in the continuing care of older people, and more often than not are responsible for delegating care to a largely unqualified staff of care assistants. Registered nurses are responsible for supervising care assistants and ensuring that they are competent to take on any delegated tasks; they should not be expected to work beyond their level of competence. Managers should provide a job description which outlines the scope of their responsibilities. At minimum they will require training in health and safety procedures as well as maintaining confidentiality. Aspects of care specific to older people would form the basis of a simple training programme.

If the manager is educated to specialist practice standard, then much of this could be achieved on the job, in a systematic way and over a period of time. National Vocational Qualifications (NVQs or in Scotland SCOTVECs), and the newer General (G) NVQ in Health and Social Care, enable people without qualifications to acquire them, through demonstration of competence at work.

There are a number of diferent levels of competence for NVQs. Level 2 covers basic skills, and it is at this level that most care assistants are expected to work. Level 3 extends beyond this basic level to include the ability to contribute to planning care.

In order to achieve an NVQ, the carer will need to register with an awarding body, which may be a local further education (FE) college or a department of nursing in a college of higher education. On payment of the registration fee, the carer will receive the appropriate assessment documents and access to a work-based assessor. In the care home setting, the assessor will be a first-level qualified nurse, who has had additional training in order to fulfill this role. Qualified nurses with a specialist qualification in the care of older people, together with a teaching qualification, can play a key role in training and supporting care assistants. In this way the care worker learns best practice from an expert, and contributes to the overall maintenance of quality care. In turn this enhances the reputation of the home.

The address of a local NVQ awarding body can be obtained through a job centre or by contacting a local college of further education. Some FE colleges offer study days and short courses which introduce the activities and knowledge required for an NVQ. There are also open or distance learning packages, whereby those people who feel sufficiently confident and motivated to work alone, can do so at home in their own time.

The following topics are suggested as the basis for an in-service training programme for care assistants:

- fire prevention and procedure in the event of fire,
- home safety and first aid,
- confidentiality,
- giving personal care,
- sensory loss and communication,
- prevention of pressure sores,
- manual handling,
- normal ageing,
- therapeutic approaches in caring for residents with dementia,
- care of the dying resident,
- providing recreational activities,
- nutrition and feeding strategies,
- meeting religious and cultural needs, and anti-discriminatory practices, and
- elimination and continence care.

The teaching/learning process in later life

Learning can be defined as 'those processes leading to relatively permanent changes in potential for performance as a consequence of experience' (Shea, 1991). 'Processes' would include such things as attention, ability to think, reason and remember. 'Relatively permanent' suggests that the change continues over a period. 'Potential for performance' suggests that, once learning has taken place, the response is different. 'Experience' can be formal, as in a planned teaching session, or informal, whereby it can happen at any time in the course of daily living. It is the formal experience of the learning process that is the concern of this section.

Older people have more chronic conditions and multiple pathology and are major users of the health and social care services. A person's ability to maintain some independence as a result of behaviour which maximises their state of well-being and ability to care for themselves contributes to autonomy and a sense of self-esteem. It is also desirable in terms of increased effectiveness.

Older people can, and want, to learn more about their health status (Pascucci, 1992). Health education and health teaching for older adults is not always viewed as a priority. This is possibly as a result of ageist beliefs, for example, that older people are unable to learn or that it is too late to make any difference to inevitable decline. Current research suggests that older people continue to learn right up to the end of their lives, so long as disease does not interfere with the 'processes' integral to learning already described.

However, biological and socio-cultural age changes do affect the learning process so that, if teaching strategies are to be successful, they must be modified to take account of these differences. Age changes in the central nervous system, and decreased blood flow to the brain, slow the rate of information processing, reaction time and response rates. Short-term memory, now increasingly known as secondary memory, is also affected in that the laying down of information in the memory store, and recalling it when required to do so, is less efficient. Continuing opportunities to utilise and rehearse what is remembered have been found to be a significant factor in preserving ability to remember (Holland and Rabbitt, 1991).

Sensory impairments such as changes in hearing and sight must be considered in the delivery of a teaching session and the design of any supporting materials. Musculo-skeletal limitations may affect the person's ability to perform a new skill. To compensate for these changes, the nurse should adopt a slower pace, allowing time for questions from the learner. Small amounts of information which are repeated frequently, are more likely to be assimilated. One to three concepts relating to a subject is thought to be sufficient for a single session (Weinrich and Boyd, 1992). Verbal communication can be reinforced with written material. Print size of 16–18 point is recommended.

Instructions requiring the holding and manipulation of ideas in the head tend to put older people at a disadvantage. When this is unavoidable, instructions should proceed step by step. Decreased ability to concentrate can be countered by reducing external stimuli, such as surrounding conversations and noise from radio and television. The client's own room or home is preferable for one to one teaching. The older person is less able to think in abstracts, so everyday examples should be used to illustrate abstract information. For example water pressure in a garden hose could be likened to blood pressure, in order to describe the dangers of hypertension. Decreased visuo-spatial ability complicates an older person's ability to learn a new skill, so that more time is needed for demonstration and practice. A good light without glare will help compensate for poor sight.

Older people will have had shorter periods of formal education. Eight years of schooling is likely to be the norm for the majority. Also teaching methods were much more didactic, with little informal two-way communication between pupil and teacher. Continued encouragement from the nurse is essential to overcome societal views and beliefs from older people themselves, who may feel that they are beyond formal learning. It can be pointed out to them that they have had almost a lifetime of learning from experience and that this is to their advantage.

The stages of the nursing process offer a useful framework for organising and giving a teaching session. Assessment will cover the cognitive, sensory and attitudinal aspects already discussed, together with the person's health beliefs, existing knowledge on the topic and its relevance to their cultural values. If the desired change in behaviour is incompat-ible with religious beliefs, food choices and socio-cultural values, it is likely to be a waste of time. Planning will involve setting goals and choosing an appropriate method and location. It will help if the person's main carer is also present, so as to be able to encourage and support him through the learning experience. In the community, this could be a support worker or significant other, and in a care home, the older person's key worker.

Implementation is followed by evaluation as to whether the learner has understood, retained or demonstrated the desired material or skill. Clues about the effectiveness of the teaching can be gained from the type of questions the learner asks, as well as statements and comments. New skills can be assessed by observation by both nurse, significant others and key workers.

Group teaching in care homes

Residents' meetings can be used to determine their health teaching requirements, or alternatively through a simple large print questionnaire. Ormson (1987) describes a success story which should give inspiration to nurses who wish to begin health teaching but are not sure on how are where to start. Residents chose topics relating to their chronic conditions, about which most had little or no understanding. Sessions were kept short (15–20 minutes), and visual and auditory material was presented using an overhead projector and a sound system. Of course, this equip-ment may not be available to small homes and staff will have to rely on their own resourcefulness to present material which is accessible to resi-dents with sight and hearing deficits. Opportunity for discussion was an integral part of each session and large print handouts were distributed for participants to read at their leisure.

Burdette (1993) describes a similar experience with an informal educa-tion programme which started as a result of the author being asked to advise on the prevention of chronic constipation. This led to topics such as hypertension, pain, stress, loss of hearing and vision, and other chronic conditions.

Guidelines for good practice
- Adopt a slower pace.
- Stick to small amounts of information and repeat it.
- Reinforce verbal communication with written material in large print.
- Pick a quiet spot with no distractions.
- Compensate for deficits in hearing and sight.
- Use everyday examples to illustrate concepts.
- Use repetition to reinforce small amounts of information.
- Allow more time for demonstration and practice when teaching new skills.
- Use suitable lighting.

Continuing educational opportunities for older people

The need for self-fulfilment continues for most people right up until the end of life itself. There have been some very successful projects in continuing care wards whereby older people have derived pleasure and satisfaction from participating in literary and artistic pursuits. There are likely to be long gaps in residents' days, and activities can maximise quality of life, by stimulating mental activity and raising morale. Activities also change the status of the individual from patient to student, thus adding variety to a potentially monotonous routine. Residents can be canvassed as to their needs at their meetings, and appropriate tutors obtained by advertising in the local newspaper.

Conclusion

Education is a key aspect of life in care homes for both the staff and the residents. Within the UKCC Code of Professional Conduct and the Post Registration Education and Practice framework, nurses who work with older people in care homes have a responsibility to maintain high standards of practice, and to develop their professional knowledge and competence. Although nurses in some care homes may face particular challenges in accessing educational courses and facilites, there are many formal and informal ways in which they can develop their knowledge and their practice. Many educational institutions now offer greater flexibility, for example with evening classes, distance learning, and accreditation for prior learning or experience. Creating a stimulating learning environment, with reflective practice and clinical supervision, can facilitate the development of all staff in the home. The residents and their families can also benefit from education, provided that this is offered in a manner which is sensitive to health status and age-related changes. A great deal of enjoyment and fulfilment can be gained from stimulating life-long learning.

Resources for continuing education and training

Age Concern Training, PO Box B96, Hammonds Yard, King Street, Huddersfield, HD1 1WT or 1268 London Road, London SW16 4ER.
Age Exchange Reminiscence Centre, 11 Blackheath Village, London SE3 9LA.
BASE (British Association for Service to the Elderly), (Wales), 4th Floor, Transport House, 1 Cathedral Road, Cardiff CF1 9SD.

Local authority health promotion departments

Organisations dedicated to a particular cause, such as Arthritis Care, or the Parkinson's Disease Society, can be approached for information and useful leaflets.

National Extension College, 18 Brooklands Avenue, Cambridge CB2 2HN.

Institute of Advanced Nursing Education, Royal College of Nursing, 20 Cavendish Square, London W1M 0AB.

Departments of nursing within universities.

Distance Learning, e.g. Open University modules: 'An Ageing Society', and 'Working with Older People' The Open University, PO. Box 188, Milton Keynes MK7 6DH.

Local further education colleges.

Training materials for carers working towards achieving vocational qualifications can be obtained from The Open College, St Paul's, 781 Wilmslow Road, Didsbury, Manchester M20 2RW.

Local careers centres

Nursing Home News (published by the Registered Nursing Homes Association).

Elderly Care (published six times per annum). Continuing education articles with accompanying assessments enable nurses to earn ten Continuing Education (CE) credits: – equivalent to one study day.

References

Burdette, C. (1993) COPE: Concerned Oldsters' Program of Education. *Geriatric Nursing*, **14** (1) 42–44.

Department of Health (1994) The Challenges to Nursing and Midwifery in the 21st Century (The Heathrow Report). London: HMSO.

Department of Health NHS and Community Care Act 1990. London: HMSO.

Eaves, K. (1988) Educational needs in the private sector. *Senior Nurse*, **8**, 2.

Holland, C.A. and Rabbitt, P.M.A., (1991) Ageing Memory: Use versus impairment. *British Journal of Psychology*, **82**, 29–38

NHS Management Executive (1993) A vision for the future. The nursing, midwifery and health visiting contribution to health and healthcare. Department of Health.

Norton, D. (1990) *The Age of Old Age*. London: Scutari Press.

Office of Population Censuses and Surveys (1993) The 1991 Census: Persons Aged 60 And Over in Great Britain. London: HMSO.

Ormson, L. (1987) Resident Talks. *Canadian Nurse*, **83**, 4, 29–31.

Pascucci, M. A. (1992) Measuring Incentives to Health Promotion in Older Adults. *Journal of Gerontological Nursing*, **18**, 3, 16–23.

Phillipson, C. and Strang, P. (1986) *Training and Education for an Ageing Society: New perspectives for the Health and Social Services*. Health Education Council.

Royal College of Nursing (1992) *A Scandal Waiting to Happen*. London: RCN.

Shea, P. (1991) Learning, Teaching and Ageing: Unpublished paper.

United Kingdom Central Council for Nursing, Midwifery and Health Visiting (1992a) Code of Professional Conduct, London: UKCC.

United Kingdom Central Council for Nursing Midwifery and Health Visiting (1992b). The Scope of Professional Practice. London: UKCC.

United Kingdom Central Council for Nursing, Midwifery and Health Visiting (1994a) The Future of Professional Practice – the Council's Standards for Education and Practice Following Registration. London: UKCC.

United Kingdom Central Council for Nursing, Midwifery and Health Visiting (1994b) Professional Conduct – Occasional Report on Standards of Nursing in Nursing Homes. London: UKCC.

Weinrich, S.P and Boyd, M. (1992) Education in the Elderly. *Journal of Gerontological Nursing*, **18**, 1.

Further reading

Weinrich, S.P., Boyd, M. and Nussbaum, J. (1989) Continuing Education. Adapting Strategies to Teach the Elderly. *Journal of Gerontological Nursing*, **5**, 11, 17–22.

Denham, M. J. (ed.) (1991) (ed) *Care of the Long-Stay Elderly Patient* (2nd edition). London: Chapman & Hall.

10

Communication

Jim Marr

Introduction

How many of us remember the times during our student nurse training when the ward was quiet and the work up to date? Sister would appear and ask us to 'go and speak to the patients'. Off we would go, rather reluctantly, and seek out someone who was young, attractive and easy to talk to. If we had to communicate, we wanted it to be as easy as possible! Someone who was our own age, independent and, usually, the opposite sex, offered the best chance for an amusing and interesting exchange. We had things in common to discuss, perhaps shared memories and a mutual understanding of each other's experiences. Rarely would we seek out a patient who was old. Older people, generally, were more difficult to talk to and required more time and effort on our part.

Skills in communicating with patients evolve and develop through time and so it may be argued that student nurses require varied learning experiences in order to become proficient. A basic requirement of entry into nurse education is an ability to communicate, but the novice practitioner is exposed to many events and situations which are sensitive and complex, where patients are emotionally upset, and these skills are cultivated and honed during training and into registered practice. Similarly skills in communicating with older people evolve and develop with experience. As time is invested in communication with others, eventually a relationship develops which is founded on the mutual exchange between those concerned.

In this chapter, I will explore the issues around communication with older people, taking account of their special needs which are sometimes complicated by the ageing process and disease or disability. The evolution and formation of therapeutic relationships between the nurse and the older person as an integral part of continued care will also be explored.

Communication Skills

From infancy, these skills are learned firstly by observation, initially from our parents but later from our peers. At play, children can be heard enacting communication exchanges between adults - often their teacher. Skills are therefore also learned by imitation. Eventually into adolescence they are practised in a variety of settings as our social network enlarges. Sometimes, this period is also used to try out different types of anti-social behaviour, such as manipulation and sulking, in our attempts to influence others. Hopefully, into adulthood, these interpersonal skills fully evolve and the individual becomes a mature and well-balanced person – knowing themselves intimately and their effect on others. It is also hoped that the individual will thereafter become a law-abiding citizen and a responsible member of society.

Ageism in society

The society in which we live is preoccupied with youth and young people. This is partly due to the fact that younger people are seen to be avid consumers with a large disposable income. During the Thatcher era in the late 1980's, we saw the emergence of the 'Yuppie' culture where young professionals with large salaries were seduced by the media and the market forces. In the early 1990's young older people, i.e. those who were newly retired, were also seen to be a major consumer force and it was interesting to observe a rise in the advertising aimed at this group. In the main however, older people are not valued by society at large.

The Political Economy Theory of Ageing (Phillipson and Walker, 1986) explains the failure of the Government to deal with the demographic changes of the country and make special provision for the needs of the rising numbers of older people. Older people began to be perceived as a 'problem' by politicians when it was really the failure of government planning and policies that was the problem. However, this negative notion of older people has continued to permeate society and is even noted in the health and social services where high dependency and continued care services are now viewed as non-profit making and a drain on resources.

Valuing older people

The life experience, wisdom and skills of older people are a very valuable resource within our society. Throughout the twentieth century these individuals have survived major wars, poverty, deprivation, political, economic and technological changes. Modern society has been shaped by these people and they have held the belief that society would recognise their achievements and would support them in later life. Although many older people live happy, comfortable lives, for others each day brings a struggle to cope with poverty, disability and ill-health.

It should be remembered, however, that ageing is a normal process and old age should be viewed as a developmental stage of life when sacrifice, hard work and political activity may be reduced and an individual feels able to enter a period of fulfilment and happiness.

For many older people, retirement means a huge period of adjustment when they leave behind influential roles associated with employment and adapt to other roles in their life brought about by major changes such as reduced income, loss of family and friends and possibly increased dependency on outside agencies to meet their health and social needs. These major losses in their life often become a drain on previously established coping skills and some older people may find themselves overwhelmed and unable to adjust. For many, this failure to cope becomes a pathological process and results in an emotional disorder known as clinical depression. Depressive illness is identified as the major mental health problem of older age (Victor, 1991).

For many older people the loss of roles and the reduction of social stimulation may cause them to partly withdraw from society and thus they risk becoming isolated, lonely and under-stimulated (Murphy, 1982). This may result in their view of the world becoming negative and they may feel rejected, becoming bitter towards others. Thus society may withdraw from them. Disorientation and confusion may then arise due to the effects of social and sensory deprivation. Eventually this may result in the older people being referred to health and social services, often resulting in a new role as patient, client or resident. Thus the individual becomes caught up in the complicated machinery of 'care' services.

Therapeutic relationships

In all formal 'care' situations the basis of the care is centred around the ability of the carers to form a relationship with the patient/client/resident. This relationship is deemed to be therapeutic in that it is based on a mutual respect, trust, tolerance, understanding and friendliness, as are most relationships (Ironbar, 1983). However this is a 'professional' relationship and care staff are expected to invest time and effort into making it succeed as part of their normal duties. There is no room for the likes and dislikes which normally dictate the formation of a relationship; staff are paid to care for everyone. This does not mean, however, that 'favourites' do not develop as we are all human beings with different personality traits.

The therapeutic relationship usually begins on admission to the care setting although it is now becoming common practice for pre-admission visits to be carried out in an attempt to encourage early formation of such. Other organisational policies such as 'primary nursing', 'the named nurse' and 'keyworker' systems or 'patient allocation' facilitate early information-gathering and encourage the development of the relationship. Muetzel (1988) describes three components of nurse–patient relationships. These are intimacy, partnership and reciprocity, and combinations of these form the 'atmosphere', 'dynamics' and 'spirit' of any relationship, determining how successfully the individuals react together.

The formation of therapeutic relationships with older people may be quite complex as each has such a long and varied life experience and diverse needs in the care situation. Sometimes the age-gap can be difficult for younger members of staff they as may not have common interests or shared experiences, although this is not always the case as many grandparents and grandchildren have better relationships than with the middle generation. In care settings, techniques such as life-review, reminiscence therapy and care-mapping may encourage the older person to be viewed as an individual with a unique life experience. This may further relationship building.

Some studies have shown communications between nurses and older people to be brief and infrequent based mainly around nursing procedures and tasks (MacLeod-Clark, 1983). In many cases conversation is centred around closed questioning with little opportunity given for the individual to respond in detail or much time given for interacting. This was said to be a by-product of task-orientated care but others suggest that it is the nurse's way of dealing and coping with distressing situations and is a technique used to distance themselves from emotionally draining situations. In some high dependency areas it may also be a reaction to an overwhelming demand in the face of scarce resources.

For many older people, a traditional respect for medicine is demonstrated as conformity behaviour within a system where they do not expect to make decisions for themselves and it is often difficult to encourage them to make choices, even at meal-times. In day-to-day relationships this conformity may also discourage the older person from being assertive or from engaging in discussion as an equal partner. Thus the trend for 'empowerment' within the Patient's Charter may be a difficult one to encourage in services for older people.

Effective communication

Effective communication between individuals is a complex process relying on many different factors coming into play at the same time. In the health and social services it is vital that communications are effective so that individuals are fully informed and thus able to give informed consent. Much distress has been generated over the years because of poor communications and this remains the biggest source of complaints in the health service sector (Audit Commission, 1992).

All communications are a mixture of verbal and non-verbal responses and sometimes these are particularly complex with older people due to age-related changes or, as mentioned previously, their reluctance to assert themselves and ask for further information or clarification of detail. MacLeod-Clark (1991) identifies four main communication needs of older people in hospitals:

- social contact and interaction,
- explanation and confirmation,
- advice, education and support, and
- comfort and reassurance.

These are fundamental to the development of effective therapeutic relationships and yet are often overlooked when caring for older adults – perhaps a sign of the ageism in care services.

Non-verbal skills

Non-verbal communication is particularly important when caring for older people as Argyle (1978) claims that it is five times more effective than verbal communication. In institutional care settings patients/ clients/residents are onlookers for a large part of the time and, as they watch care staff at work, they continually assess and form impressions of them as individuals. Eventually they learn who to approach, and who not to, for help in meeting their needs. The initial assessment made of the care worker is to find out if the he/she is a 'good person' and it is thus important to place him/her in a social context. They will ask details of the staff member's background, family life, etc., and from this decide whether they will 'get on' together. Following this initial assessment it is then important to find out if they are a 'good nurse/professional' who is competent and reliable. Much of this information is gleaned informally from observations of interactions with others or shared amongst other patients/clients/residents as part of their assessment process.

The physical appearance of care staff is also important to older people and many feel more comfortable when staff are in some type of uniform. Marr and Matthews (1993) found that older people have fairly narrow perceptions of how nurses should look and behave, perhaps based on traditional beliefs of the role. As services and roles change over the years, their expectations may not match the reality and may require some adjustment. Much of this is formulated from their perceptions and from non-verbal communications.

All types of behaviour convey messages as do body language, facial expression and touch. These may convey to an older person much more about feelings and attitude than what is said – particularly if hearing impairment is present. Eye contact is perhaps the most important feature of facial expression and is used initially to engage someone in conversation by gaining their attention. Frequently care staff, in an effort to attract attention, are seen to invade body space by coming too close. This may appear threatening to an older person and cause them to be nervous and apprehensive. It may be better practice to touch the hand initially to engage in conversation. Failure to achieve eye contact during conversation may be interpreted as insincerity, lack of interest or mistrust and is a frequent cause of offence to older people.

Other details of body language such as posture, gestures or head-nodding add texture to communications (Peplau, 1992). This may be the first signal given about an emotional state, e.g. a stooped posture signifying depression or withdrawal. Similarly, a nurse who leans forward during conversation may appear more interested than one who slumps backwards. Gestures are also very important – especially hand signals – and these are frequently used in communications with older people to supplement speech. Head-nodding during conversation acts as an encouragement and demonstrates understanding and active listening, particularly in combination with good eye contact. A slight exaggeration of these is useful in encouraging the speech-impaired or those with expressive disorders.

Verbal skills

Verbal communication is mainly thought to be about speech. However speech can be subdivided into two main components: form and content. Content deals with what is actually being said, e.g. the topic of conversation, and form is concerned with the way it is said, e.g. pace, orientation and comprehension.

Earlier in the chapter we touched upon initial relationship-building and how difficult it can be for a younger person to find common themes to discuss with someone much older. Often in institutional care, much of the topic of conversation is mundane and meaningless and discourages meaningful communication. Listen to conversations in your own workplace and you will hear exchanges about the weather, food, appearance or physical care but very little about current affairs, or social or psychological needs. Perhaps this is part of the strategy of care staff in distancing themselves as meaningless conversation may be seen as 'safe' – no more problems or work will be generated and thus time will be spared for other activities. This may be a sign of overwhelming need in the face of scarce resources.

The form of speech is mainly concerned with voice quality, although rate and clarity of speech are also important. From early days we learn to pick up messages and meaning from the sound of a voice and increase or decreases in tone, pitch and volume can greatly vary the meaning of what is said. These skills stay with us all of our lives and are particularly important in old age especially if one is dependent on others for help in meeting fundamental needs. Unhelpful attitudes of care staff are noted not in what they say, but how it is said. Underlying messages are given and received and frequently convey authority, superiority, sarcasm and even threat. These are powerful messages and may further reinforce feelings of powerlessness, dependency and conformity in care settings.

Counselling

Despite the enormous amount of material published about counselling, there are still those who seem to believe it is a technique freely available for the enthusiastic amateur to meddle with. Skilled counselling takes many years of study and practice to achieve, and a great deal of harm may be done by meddling. It is true that many people are naturally good listeners who refrain from giving advice but there are very many individuals who seem able to advise others on a wide degree of topics whilst appearing quite uniformed themselves.

Some counselling techniques, however, are useful to use with older people to encourage effective communication (Ebersole and Hess, 1990). Open questioning which probes gently to elicit information and encourage the exploration of feelings may be used in a variety of everyday situations, e.g. when someone is relaxed in a bath. Information gathered and exchanged may be fundamental to the development of a therapeutic relationship. Similarly the technique of active listening may be equally useful and an effective skill for dealing with older people. It should be remembered that any form of close communication should be a two-way process and should be conducted in a suitable environment in a non-threatening manner.

Touch

A further powerful method of communication is through touch and this can evoke strong messages both negatively and positively. Over the last few years we have observed an upsurge of literature in the nursing journals about the use of touch, mainly concerning complementary therapies such as massage, particularly using aromatherapy oils. The value of therapeutic touch has also been discussed at length (Sayre-Adams, 1995). The use of touch in this context has further added to the skills available to nursing staff, and in many care settings it is commonplace for staff to use massage and aromatherapy as a first step to relieving pain, reducing emotional upset and for promoting rest and sleep.

Oliver and Redfern (1991) claim that nursing staff do not use effective touch when caring for older people. Much of the touch is described as instrumental, done deliberately in the performance of tasks such as dressing a wound or recording blood pressure. In continued care settings, touch may only be carried out when moving and handling individuals. Some older people may therefore suffer from touch deprivation – especially men. This is particularly unfortunate in institutional care as many older people may rarely have visits from friends or family and thus rely on care staff for stimulation in this way. It is not difficult to see how an older person may almost be encouraged to be incontinent – at least they experience touch and stimulation during 'toileting'.

Barnett (1972) identifies touch as providing comfort, relief from physical or psychological pain, and as sensory stimulation, reality orientation and sexual expression. Sometimes it can be used inappropriately, such as patting someone's head in a child-like fashion and many older people may have particular taboos about touch stemming from earlier years when society was perhaps more formal. It may be regarded as intimacy and cause offence. In modern society there are still many cultural and social rules surrounding touch and where and when it is permitted. Acceptable touch depends on age, situation, life experience and the environment. It is very important for care staff to realise cultural differences especially with touch between the opposite sexes. It is not unusual for elderly Asian women to be beaten by their husbands following a period of hospitalisation because they allowed themselves to be seen or touched by male staff.

For most older people however, touch remains a very effective method of communication – especially for those suffering from sensory impairment. It can clearly demonstrate acceptance, trust, affection and understanding and is a skill which should be cultivated and acknowledged in all care settings for the elderly. For older people with a depressive or dementing illness, touch may be the only method of effective communication.

Communication difficulties for older people

It is important to realise that not all older people are ill or disabled and many rarely need to call on health or social services, living fairly independent, comfortable lives. Those who work in care services see and deal with the small minority of ill older people and it is not difficult to begin to form the impression that old age is inevitably a time of decay and despair.

Some older people, however, do suffer from a degree of sensory impairment, related to disease or the ageing process, especially visual loss or hearing impairment. A reduction of sensory input will obviously have a great impact on the ability to communicate effectively and some older people may also suffer from expressive disorders or cognitive impairment. Changes such as these can easily result in social withdrawal, loneliness and isolation (Murphy, 1982).

For any older person in this situation, it is vital that a full assessment is made of their needs (and their abilities!) so that an individual care package can be designed with all the multi-disciplinary team working together creatively to encourage the enhancement of communication.

Visual impairment

For very many people, ageing changes within the eye begin to cause problems for them in their forties or early fifties, resulting in the need for spectacles to aid focusing for close work. In later years older people may also experience difficulty in adjusting to darkness. It is estimated that older people need 70 per cent more light than do younger people to see normally. These special difficulties often result in frequent accidents and falls, especially at night.

Visual difficulties affect communication as gestures, facial expressions and lip-reading may be misinterpreted or missed altogether and thus much of the 'social texture' during interactions is lost. Regular eye testing is therefore important in old age as other disease and disorders may have an insidious onset which is easily explained away as 'old age'.

For those older people who need to wear spectacles or use magnifying glasses, it is vital that these are looked after carefully by nursing staff and are not forgotten or left in bedside lockers during the day when the older person is up and about. They should be cleaned regularly and protected from scratches when not being used. In many institutions these personal effects are marked for easy identification and this can be done discreetly using a denture marking kit rather than adhesive tape being wrapped around the object.

Communication with visually impaired older people can be enhanced with thoughtfulness and good practice from carers:

- Ensure that areas are appropriately lit.
- Avoid vividly patterned or geometric floor coverings.
- Maintain a stable, familiar environment which is safe from accidental injury.
- Encourage the use of spectacles and other equipment.

- Re-assess these regularly and treat them with care.
- Provide large-print reading materials, radio, talking books, tapes, etc.
- Use environmental aids such as clear labelling, colour coding, large clocks, etc.
- Introduce yourself before speaking and use touch to attract attention.
- Face the person at a level which encourages eye contact.
- Spend time interacting and encourage leisure activities.

Hearing impairment

Problems with hearing also become more common in older age groups although some minor problems such as ear-wax can easily be overlooked and cause unnecessary suffering.

The most common impairment due to ageing is the gradual loss of higher pitched sounds, although sound distortion and tinnitis are also common. Ageing changes within the ear may also affect balance thus increasing the likelihood of falls.

As with visual impairment, hearing loss is frequently slow and imperceptible, the older person frequently denying its existence and blaming others for muttering or speaking quietly. Many older people become suspicious, imagining that others are excluding them purposely and a degree of paranoia may develop. Even after hearing loss has been identified, some older people may refuse to wear a hearing aid. This may be because of the perceived stigma of disability or because aids amplify all sound and this may prove to be intolerable for some. It should also be remembered that a hearing aid will only help those people with conductive deafness and requires a period of perseverance, adjustment and skill to operate successfully. Effective use relies on proper care and maintenance which many older people are unable to achieve. These skills are therefore desirable in those nursing staff caring for them.

Effective communication with hearing impaired older adults can be encouraged with skill and good practice. Points for consideration are as follows:

- Ensure that the ear and auditory canal are free from obstruction.
- Eliminate background noise as much as possible.
- Check and maintain hearing aids.
- Supplement oral communication with other methods, e.g. writing, pictures, signs and gestures.
- Face the person directly to achieve eye contact and enable lip-reading.
- Do not cover the mouth or turn away when speaking.
- Speak slowly and clearly without exaggeration or shouting.
- Check understanding frequently and rephrase if necessary.
- Stick to the main subject without unnecessary detail.

Speech impairment

The most common reason for speech impairment in older people is usually a result of a cerebrovascular accident (CVA). For some people, however, the reason may be due to hearing loss, isolation or poorly fitting dentures.

Speech impairment can have a disastrous effect on communication, causing great frustration to the victim as well as the listener. Isolation is common as others give up communicating because it becomes too difficult or tedious. Following a CVA it is important to identify whether the impairment is one of two types of dysphasia: receptive or expressive. Receptive dysphasia means that the person cannot understand language whilst expressive dysphasia means that there is still an understanding of verbal and written communication, but an inability to organise ideas into words, and thus expression is lost (Ebersole and Hess, 1990). This is particularly frustrating for the individual as understanding is intact but response is impaired. Many are subjected to infantile communication from others, or recognise frustration and annoyance. Time and patience are vital if interactions are to be meaningful and therapeutic. Sometimes other factors such as memory loss, disorientation, emotional disorder or loss of concentration, may also complicate communication following a CVA.

For those caring for an older person with speech impairment, good practice is essential. The following points should be considered:

- Be patient and give plenty time for a response.
- Treat the person as normal, addressing them by name and using touch skills.
- Ensure good eye contact.
- Speak slowly, using gestures and signs where appropriate.
- Phrase questions to encourage a simple response.
- Encourage the use of other aids such as signs, pictures etc.
- Do not pretend to understand if you don't – ask them to repeat or rephrase.
- Pay attention to non-verbal cues such as behaviour and facial expression.
- Avoid long interactions which become tiring.
- Encourage and explain skills to friends and relatives.
- Encourage normal interests, hobbies and activities.
- Give praise, support and positive feedback.

Cognitively-impaired older people

For many nursing staff, communication with those individuals who have a dementing illness offers most challenge and the special skills required appear to evade them. Features of dementia such as memory loss, disorientation and behavioural changes have a great impact on effective communication and the progression of the condition makes it more and more difficult. It is therefore vital that much information is gathered and recorded about the person as an individual to give guidance and clues to needs and desires later, as the older person experiences difficulty in expressing themselves and in understanding others

In the early stages of dementia, insight into the condition and its effects frequently causes depression and isolation in the individual resulting from lack of confidence or low self-esteem. Effective communication and the development of a therapeutic relationship is vital and the mutual trust and understanding will serve as an investment later as deterioration continues.

Useful therapeutic techniques such as reality orientation, reminiscence and validation therapy have been explained elsewhere in the text and nursing staff should be skilled in their use, knowing when and where to apply them (and when not to!). As deterioration continues there comes a time when re-orientation is not possible and indeed may further distress the older person. The skilled nurse must know when and how to alter communication to focus on the emotional state rather than dwell on the meanings of the words used.

In later stages, non-verbal communication becomes particularly important and meaning may be gleaned from behaviour and past experiences with the individual. The skilled use of touch, facial expression, gestures, eye contact, tone of voice and posture on the nurse's part may greatly enhance and encourage effective communications (Beck and Heacock, 1988).

Communication with cognitively impaired older people should include the following features:

- Address the person using their preferred name.
- Obtain their attention before speaking.
- Introduce yourself.
- Look directly at them, using touch where appropriate and a pleasant facial expression.
- Maintain a calm and reassuring voice, rephrasing where necessary.
- Be simple, but respectful, and reinforce with non-verbal cues.
- Give time to respond, attempt to elicit feelings and understand emotions.
- If there is a lack of response or co-operation, return when they are more amenable.
- Encourage the use of reminiscence, reality orientation and validation techniques.
- Give simple, relevant information and encourage simple choices.
- Be flexible and creative in all interactions and care.

Conclusion

In all interaction and communications with older people, it should be remembered that older people have a life-time of experience on which to draw and therefore quickly identify insincerity and patronising behaviour in others. Negative attitudes and poor communication skills are difficult to disguise and many older people are expert at assessing others. In continuing care, patients/residents/clients spend much time watching and listening to staff when they are unaware and off-guard. In this way they make assumptions and reach conclusions about who to approach for help and advice and who not to. Similarly decisions are reached about their investments in relationships with members of staff and choices are made about who to trust and who to avoid.

Towards the end of life, social interactions are reduced through choice and only meaningful relationships are continued. Older people may be seen to withdraw and spend less effort in exchanges with others, appearing preoccupied in their own thoughts and day-dreams. At this time it is often noticeable that they seem to make choices about when, and with whom, to communicate. Perhaps this stage is an indication of which nurses have communicated effectively and shown genuine care, thus achieving a meaningful and therapeutic relationship. Perhaps it is these relationships which the older person values most and chooses to maintain?

References

Argyle, M. (1978) *The Psychology of Interpersonal Behaviour*. Harmondsworth: Penguin.

Audit Commission (1992) *Making Time for Patients: a Handbook for Ward Sisters*. London: HMSO.

Barnett, K. (1972) 'A Survey of the Current Utilisation of Touch by Health Team Personnel with Hospitalized Patients'. *International Journal of Nursing Studies*, **9**, 195–209.

Beck, K and Heacock, P. (1988) Nursing Interventions for Patients with Alzheimer's Disease. *Nursing Clinics of North America*, **23**, 95–121.

Ebersole, P. and Hess, P. (1990) *Toward Healthy Aging: Human Needs and Nursing Response*. Toronto: CV Mosby Co.

Ironbar, N. (1983) *Self Instruction in Psychiatric Nursing*. Eastbourne: Balliere Tindall.

MacLeod-Clark, J. (1983) Nurse-Patient Communication: an Analysis of Conversations from Surgical Wards. In J. Wilson-Barnett, (ed.) *Nursing Research: Ten Studies in Patient Care*. Chichester: John Wiley.

MacLeod-Clark, J. (1991) Communicating with Elderly People' in S. Redfern (ed.) *Nursing Elderly People*. London: Churchill Livingstone.

Marr, J. and Matthews, T. (1993) Change of a Dress. *Nursing Standard*, **19**, August 25, 48–49.

Muetzel, P. (1988) Therapeutic Nursing in A. Pearson, (ed.) *Primary Nursing*. Kent: Croom Helm Ltd.

Murphy, E. (1982) Social Origins of Depression in Old Age, *British Journal of Psychiatry*, **141**, 135

Oliver, S. and Redfern, S. (1991) Interpersonal Communication Between Nurses and Elderly Patients. *Journal of Advanced Nursing*, **16**, 30–38.

Peplau, H. (1992) *Interpersonal Relationships in Nursing*. Basingstoke: Macmillan Press Ltd.

Phillipson, C. and Walker, A. (1986) *Ageing and Social Policy*. Aldershot: Gower.

Sayre-Adams, J. (1995) *Therapeutic Touch*. Edinburgh: Churchill Livingstone.

Victor, C. (1991) *Health and Health Care in Later Life*. Buckingham: Open University Press.

Clinical Matters

11

Mental Health

Liz Matthew

Introduction

Demographic changes mean that there are now more people enjoying the later years of their life, but there are also a substantial number of older people who will experience mental illness. Identifying exact figures of those who experience mental illness is difficult for five main reasons:

1. There are various definitions of what is old. Some studies use a baseline of 60 years, others 65, 75 and 85. This makes it difficult to compare like with like in order to produce general prevalence statistics.
2. Mental illnesses are not mutually exclusive, for example some people will experience dementia and depression, so it is not possible to provide a linear calculation by adding up the totals for individual diagnoses.
3. Not all episodes of mental illness are recorded, only those in contact with formal agencies. Although it is more likely that cases of dementia will be recorded, depression for example may be more widespread than the figures suggest.
4. Diagnostic criteria may vary and their application is subjective.
5. All statistics are dated to some extent because of the time lapse between collecting and publishing data. Statistics thus only provide 'snapshots' which are bound to be retrospective.

In addition, problems may occur in accurately diagnosing mental illness in older people due to a lack of clarity of their role in society (Kay et al., 1964). If older people are expected to be isolated and withdrawn for example, then a diagnosis of depression might go unrecognised. Conversely a more flamboyant person who refuses to adopt a passive role, may be labelled as demonstrating bizarre behaviours that could be seen to be symptomatic of other forms of mental illness.

Entering a care home

The move may be triggered more by the needs of the carer than the resident. If a carer is faced with constant sleep disruptions, dealing with behavioural problems, or the demands of providing 24-hour care, then pressure on the carer can result in emotional and physical distress, both to themselves and other family members It is unlikely that individuals will have had a real choice in whether or not to enter a home. They may be unable to support themselves physically by carrying out the normal functions of everyday life. There may not be family or friends who can, or are willing to, provide support in a meaningful or practical way.

The individual may no longer be able to call upon the resources which make up care in the community either because of limitations or priorities in budgets or because with the onset of mental ill-health they may not be deemed capable of looking after themselves. In effect there can be little real choice.

Part of the social world of the older person, like that of people at any age, involves making active choices of who we want to share our lives with. It is certain that in a care home intimate moments of life will be shared with strangers. For those with mental health problems there are particular challenges. Examples include a depressed person who could be labelled as anti-social because they do not spontaneously join in a group; an agitated person who needs constant re-assurance; or the widow who, following bereavement, may seem unfriendly or with-drawn, but who is only adjusting to the loss of their spouse.

Despite this, care homes offer a positive option for many with mental health needs. A care home can provide a safe and secure environment. With plenty of social contact, loneliness and isolation can be less prob-lematic. There is less concern about everyday finance and housekeeping, and most importantly, there would be easy access to nursing and medical support.

Homes that provide for those who have mental health needs must expect challenging behaviour amongst the residents. It can be difficult at times to balance rights and risks both for the individual and for the community living in the home. How do you balance such a situation? In the first place there needs to be an acceptance of so-called 'disruptive' or 'challenging' behaviour. Managers and owners will be aware of the like-lihood of such behaviour from assessments made before the client moves into the home, and they will also need to understand that as people grow old some are likely to develop mental health care needs.

It is pointless to expect the older person to exhibit the stereotyped 'serene', behaviour some expect of an older person. It is unrealistic, for example, to expect them to spend the rest of their lives sitting quietly in a corner. It is important then to understand what mental illness is, and the behaviours associated with it.

Common mental illnesses experienced by the older person

Depression

Depression is believed to be the most common mental health problem in the total population. However it is estimated that approximately 11–14 per cent of older people exhibit the symptoms of depression, although only 1–2 per cent can be considered severely affected (DoH, 1994). It has been suggested that as many as three in four cases of depression are neither recognized nor treated (Davidson et al., 1994). The term depression is used widely, but clinical depression is qualitatively different from being sad, weepy or miserable.

The causes of depression may be *psychological*, with some individuals more vulnerable than others. They may be *biological*, (chemical imbalances in the body). They may be *environmental*, as a result of poor social conditions, or distressing situations. A loss of some kind may be a cause, such as bereavement, or a traumatic event such as retirement.

Depression can be divided into two main categories external and internal but these are not mutually exclusive.

Frequent causes of external depression are:

- psychological problems (e.g. staff expectations to do things of which the older person is not capable);
- bereavement;
- loss of status or self-esteem (e.g. giving up independent living to enter residential care);
- poverty or financial loss;
- breakdown of relationships;
- loneliness and illness; and
- the side effects of using many different drugs.

Those for internal depression are:

- hereditary susceptibility;
- hormonal imbalances or disturbances;
- changes in brain chemistry; and
- severe physical illness.

Other factors which can have an effect are:

- lack of friends;
- loneliness;
- widowhood;
- recent death and accidents amongst relatives and friends; and
- moving into a care home.

Negative life events are not the only factors contributing to the onset of depression; physical factors also have their place. For example, illnesses such as influenza, shingles, and urinary tract infections, seem to contribute to depressive disorders, particularly in older people who already have a low self-esteem.

The more severe forms of depression have clear symptoms and can be detected reliably. The individual often becomes clearly agitated and may demonstrate behaviour such as restless pacing, clinging, or begging for help which creates irritation in those around them.

Because depression is a more or less universal experience there may be an unclear dividing line between the milder forms of depressive illness and normality. This is compounded by the fact that being 'sad' is often seen as a natural result of growing old. It is not surprising then that depression can be ignored.

For older people the presentation of depression is not always as identifiable as that in a younger person. For example due to problems of multiple pathology, symptoms of depression may be missed by the unskilled practitioner.

Many depressed older people present with multiple symptoms, i.e.:

- anxiety;
- becoming easily upset and moved to tears;
- expressing feelings of guilt, low self-esteem, helplessness and hopelessness;
- loss of interest in previous, and current, activities;
- suicidal tendencies, which may or may not be openly expressed;
- unable to perform social functions, which they have previously managed;
- may complain of varied somatic symptoms such as headache, chest pains, etc.;
- in some cases hypochondriasis;
- loss of appetite, and subsequent weight loss; and
- constipation.

Depression may profoundly affect communication, in particular the individual's motivation to communicate. This is likely to include both initiation of conversation and response to it. They may talk in a lowered tone with no variation and no expression. This may create an impression of inability to communicate when in fact time is needed to express thoughts and feelings. In the absense of such opportunities, frustration is likely to be experienced and may result in the individual being labelled as difficult or anti-social. Ultimately this will increase any feelings of isolation.

Confusional states

Confusion can be defined as the inability to think with normal clarity and coherence. There are many causes of such states, for example anxiety, psychological disorders or simply lack of attention. The word 'confusion' is often used loosely to describe the faulty behaviour of older people with mental illness, for example frequent disorientation and the inability to recognise companions. Sometimes, however, the word is used to describe the disease which gives rise to the symptoms. These symptoms are characteristic of a number of diseases which may be short-term and reversible or long-term and irreversible.

Distinguishing between someone who is not thinking clearly and someone who cannot think clearly is important. We should be concerned with how people reason, and not with how they act. Confusion is about problems with thought processes, not behaviour. For example communication problems could be the result of a sudden loss of hearing, due to a hearing-aid malfunction, or a lack of sleep, a long journey to hospital, or a noisey and unfriendly environment. All of these factors can contribute to an inability to concentrate and respond to relatively simple questions.

Confusional states are recognised by their suddenness, with often quite marked changes in the person's behaviour. This can be erratic and is often worse at night. The effects are displays of fear and anxiety, and conversation is likely to be incoherent. Attention and concentration are inhibited and cognitive function is impaired.

The causes of confusion are usually physical and are quite distinct from those of a mental health problem. Provided that the cause is detected it is very responsive to treatment, however in cases of rapid onset of actuate/toxic confusional states, these are highly indicative of underlying symptoms and the need for prompt investigation. Heart disease and infections especially of the chest and urinary tract are probably the most common causes in old age. Side effects of drugs can also be responsible, for example those for treatment of Parkinson's disease and depression. It is particularly important that the appropriate tests are carried out to identify the cause, and ensure the appropriate treatment.

Anxiety states

A recent study suggested that the prevalence of anxiety states in older people was between 2.2 per cent and 11.7 per cent (Lindesay et al. 1989). It also found that although such disorders are fairly common they are rarely referred for specialist help Anxiety states are often ignored in older people because there is a misguided assumption that it is an inevitable part of getting old, and secondly that it has a lesser impact on this age group. Murphy (1992) found that neither of these assumptions have any statistical basis.

Anxiety can been described as diffuse apprehension that is vague in nature and is associated with feelings of uncertainty and helplessness often occurring as a result of a threat to one's self-esteem or identity. Although a natural defensive behaviour, it becomes a problem when it takes over the individual's everyday life. Phobias and panic attacks are included in this category.

A phobia is a persistent fear of an object, or a situation that presents no actual danger, or where there is a slight risk, but this is magnified out of proportion. For example with agoraphobia the resident may be frightened to go out. There may be some predisposing factors involved, such as a fear of falling or the fact that they have got out of the habit and feel insecure outside.

Ageing itself brings with it many stresses. For example, a fear of falling may result in personally imposed restricted movement, both indoors and out. This would restrict anxiety and may be considered a successful strategy. Such behaviour would lead to isolation and immobility which clearly needs to be identified and resolved. Sometimes this is more evident in younger people because assumptions may be made about the reasons for older people being housebound. It is important that assumptions are not made about what is acceptable in the behaviour of older people.

Anxiety brings with it other physiological effects such as 'palpitations', 'butterflies in the stomach' and 'dizziness' and care staff should be aware of the implications of such descriptions.

Dementia

The word dementia has been described as a syndrome characterised by a decline in previously acquired educational, occupational or social capabilities. Difference in behaviour can include: forgetfulness, confusion, a change in emotion, or the loss of ability to control toilet functions. (Gidley and Shears, 1988).

The number of people with dementia in the UK has been estimated currently to be around 600 000 (about 70 per cent of these cases will be diagnosed as Alzheimer's disease). It is primarily recognized as a disease of older age. For instance the prevalence of dementia in the total population is less than 0.1 per cent for the age group 40–65. From the ages 65–70 this has increased to 2 per cent, and for 70–80 year olds 5 per cent. For the over 80's the figure is nearer 20 per cent (Alzheimer's Disease Society, 1994).

Alzheimer's disease

This is the most common form of dementia and was first described at the turn of the century. It is characterized by the development of large numbers of abnormal structures in the brain, which are only visible under the microscope. These disturb the connections between neighbouring nerve cells and progressively impair the brain's ability to function as a whole. The increase of these 'plaques' and 'tangles' may eventually spread to other areas of the brain.

The onset of the illness can be divided into three stages. The first stage is difficult to recognise in the beginning as it is characterised by failing memory (Sim, Turner and Smith, 1966) and muddled interpretation of the tasks of everyday life. There may also be signs of agitation and restlessness, although in some cases apathy may be displayed from the very beginning (Sjogren, Sjogren and Lindgren, 1952).

In the second stage there is increased deterioration of the motor functions which result in difficulties with: speech, swallowing, and co-ordination (Pearce and Miller, 1973).

In the third or terminal stage the individual often becomes bedridden and develops problems of both bladder and bowel control. He or she may exhibit grasping and groping actions, along with sucking reflexes. In the final stages there is rapid body wasting, despite a normal appetite.

The Royal College of Physicians and British Geriatrics Society (1992) estimate that there are now just under half a million long-term care places for elderly people in the UK, of which only 10 per cent or so are NHS beds. The remainder are in local authority residential care homes, and privately run nursing homes. Of these it is estimated that approximately 80 per cent of the current nursing home population have dementia (Capewell, Primrose and MacIntyre, 1986).

Other dementias

Multi-infarct dementia may occur alone, or in combination with Alzheimer's disease. Infarction, or death of brain tissue results when small blood vessels in the brain burst (haemorrhagic infarction) or are blocked by clots (thromboembolic infarction).

The onset can be sudden or gradual but typically progresses in a step-wise fashion, in which mental function declines and then stabilises or in some instances improves for a time, but only to deteriorate at some later point. Early in the disease there is a greater degree of awareness of disability than say in Alzheimer's disease and a relative preservation of the personality.

People with Parkinson's disease can experience intellectual impair-ment in the later stages of the disease. If dementia occurs it is often mild at the onset but tends to become progressively worse.

Huntington's chorea is an inherited degenerative brain disease due to a dominant gene, meaning that one half of all offspring of an affected indi-vidual will develop the disease. This is characterized by rapid involun-tary jerky movements and dementia beginning in adult life, and is progressive in nature.

Pick's disease is a rare degenerative disease of the brain which in some families has a genetic origin. Particular areas of the brain degenerate, specifically those of the frontal and temporal lobes. Symptoms include a change in personality which may lead to inappropriate or inhibited behaviour.

Those with Down's syndrome often develop Alzheimer-like dementia in middle age. It is characterised by severe mental retardation as well as physiological defects. The incidence of impaired intellectual function amongst those people with Aids has also become increasingly apparent. Recent memory decline, problem-solving inefficiency, and speech patterns have been recognised as early indicators of Aids-related dementia.

In Diffuse Lewy Body disease there is an abnormal accumulation of the protein ubiquitin which normally acts to protect cells from damage. The onset and progression of symptoms is variable. Some closely resemble those of Alzheimer's disease and others those of Parkinson's disease. However, a characteristic feature of this dementia is the early appearance of superimposed confusional states. There is also evidence that other mental functions, for example attention span, are more impaired in Diffuse Lewy Body disease than in typical Alzheimer's disease, or typical Parkinson's disease.

Creutzfeldt–Jacob disease is relatively rare. The gene from the prion protein has been identified and occurs in all types of trans-missible dementias; however, a minority of cases have an inherited form of the disease. The disease has a long latent period and trans-mission probably requires direct inoculation with infected tissue. Characteristics include behavioural disturbance and sudden spasmodic jerking movements. It has an insidious onset, but a rapidly progressive course.

Dementia differs from the other illnesses in that it is an organic disease of the brain which causes brain failure, rather than being an affective disorder which primarily disturbs emotion.

Managing dementia

Although dementia is incurable, it is not unmanageable. Many text-books stress the slow break down of identity and personality, and its devastating effects. It is, however, more productive to recognise dementia as a disability, and consequently the effect it has on the individual results from the quality of care which they receive. This gives a more psychosocial emphasis rather than a biological one.

A useful start is to try to see life from the client's point of view. Tom Kitwood, a psychologist specialising in dementia, uses the term 'personhood' which emphasises the need for every individual to be understood. The social psychology of every aspect of a person's daily life identifies the need for those who care for them to be able to relate and communicate, and give a response that is both helpful and enabling. The individual within a care home, despite having many people around, may still feel lonely, insecure, powerless and very frightened. They may display these feelings by becoming angry, and nurses often find it difficult to interpret the meaning behind these behaviours. As Kitwood and Bredin (1992) state, if you were that person:

> You'd want them to try to understand your language because you have such difficulties with theirs. We care best when we remember that each individual is a person and needs to be treated as such in order to be all that they can be.

It is important to remember that in the case of dementia those mental functions that fail are generally those to do with thought and memory, whilst feelings and sociability are not always as seriously affected.

When working with an older person who has dementia it helps to view behaviour in a positive way. A full assessment of the situation and consideration of the various options and strategies for care is required. It is important that all members of the care team are consistent with their approach, but yet are flexible enough to change strategy if the first option proves unsuccessful.

A problem-solving approach can also be useful employing the following four stages:

- Define what the problem is, and more importantly for whom it is a problem.
- Identify what are the possible causes, both internal and external.
- Be clear how the situation will be managed.
- Implement the plan, evaluate it, and amend it as appropriate.

Remember that it is the things that older people can no longer do that are most problematic for them. It is therefore important that the carer has the skills to enable them to facilitate these major adjustments.

Skills of assessment

Assessment of the older person concerns mental and physical health, and the way this is affected by their social circumstances. It should be a joint exercise by the home care team, as well as the wider team which may include the GP, community psychiatric nurse, social worker, geriatrician, and psycho-geriatrician as well as involvement from friends and relatives. It includes the expressed and felt needs of the individual and aims to enhance decision-making to improve or maintain positive mental health.

By consulting widely, a care plan will take into account an individual's previous health and social circumstances, as well as their personal history. By establishing empathy with the older person it is possible to help them recognise their anxiety about the nature of the intervention that is planned, and they can ensure that any plan will be jointly negotiated.

Assessment is an essential tool for clarifying impairment, describing strengths and needs, as well as underpinning therapy. It should not be confused with diagnostic testing, although testing may be one of its elements. Assessment will enable staff to analyse function, identify targets for intervention, develop care plans, monitor change and plan the delivery of care.

For this reason the single most important issue for care staff is a clear accurate and detailed assessment of the individuals in their charge. There needs to be a clear recognition of each client as a unique individual. This will require a close understanding and knowledge of their background in both a physical, psychological, mental, social and spiritual context.

An effective assessment is based on accurate knowledge and information, so in order to be of value it will require an awareness of as much background information as possible on the part of the staff. This means not only talking to the client but also to other staff, relatives, and professionals who would have been in contact with them in the past.

Without assessment any judgements made would be subjective and would be open to all kinds of misinterpretation. With older people this is particularly important because of common stereotypes about the lack of potential for improvement, and so by implication the lack of value of subsequent interventions.

The nurse has a particular role in assessment. The Royal College of Nursing (1993) suggests this involves four principles, namely:

- selecting the right assessment tools for the job;
- good interpersonal skills and relationships;
- where to make the assessment; and
- identifying individual's needs, strengths and assets upon which to plan nursing intervention.

The Royal College of Nursing's guide to assessment (1993) also provides some guidance on how to undertake assessment, suggesting that the nurse:

> **interviews:** gathering information from the individuals and significant others;
> **observes:** the individual, their environment and looks retrospectively at past life events;
> **examines:** the physical changes and mental processes that may indicate problems with lifestyle.

The guidelines also emphasise that assessment is an ongoing, continuous process that aims to identify positive factors that can be used as a stepping stone for further care planning.

It also suggests that the main area that nurses need to consider are: mood, cognitive abilities and behaviour and what is 'normal'. An individual's mood relates to the way in which they feel at a particular time in a given situation. Cognition relates to understanding and knowing what is going on around us and being able to respond appropriately to this information. Finally behaviour relates to the way in which we respond to a given situation. It includes the way in which individuals conduct themselves, what they will do or how they will act using both physical and mental energy.

During assessment it is important to examine mental state, particularly levels of consciousness, thought and speech, orientation and memory. Behaviour should include both the problem and clues to it. Social and biographical factors, and personal and professional perspectives are also important (Royal College of Nursing, 1993).

Assessment can be enhanced by the use of assessment models, which generally involve the use of manuals for testing, etc. These can be valuable in defining a baseline against which subsequent assessments can be measured. Tests are available for checking memory, communication, mobility, personality and mental health, personal adjustment and cognitive functioning.

Models of assessment

In order for the nurse to achieve a deeper understanding of the older person and the dichotomies of strength/frailty, dependence/independence, a wider approach to assessment may be necessary.

Bromley (1978) suggests a psychological case-history approach that draws upon the language and context of everyday life. This would include relatives, and other carers in order to provide another dimension to such observations. It is designed to achieve a deeper understanding of the individual, particularly the complex mixture of frailty and strength, dependence and independence seen in old age

Short symptom measures are very useful to monitor signs of change in psychological distress. The symptom rating test (SRT) (Kellner and Sheffield, 1973) is sensitive to symptom fluctuations and has component subscales measuring anxiety, depression, somatic symptoms and inadequacy. In particular the importance of commonly held views should not be under-estimated. For example, older people may be more inclined than younger people to express life satisfaction. This cannot be viewed in isolation as it has been established that older people may well have lower expectations than younger members of society. This view has been shown to be particularly relevant to women.

Physical assessment

The physical needs of older people need to be addressed in a pro-active and positive way, thus ensuring that at any age the person will receive immediate and effective treatment for their medical condition, thus improving their quality of life; if they are in pain they need to be treated.

Many older people may have multiple pathology, which can make assessment complex. In addition physical illness may be confused with the manifestations of mental ill health.

Due to the insidious onset of some physical problems, the older person may have become accustomed to their particular state of health and in some cases lowered function so much so that they themselves may not complain of any problems or unpleasant symptoms. Due to delays in treatment these may become more marked and pronounced. Older people are more prone to altered presentation of illness when there is more than one system affected (Arie, 1981).

Psychological assessment

It is only recently that the mental health issues of older people have been fully recognised and that an expectancy of proper diagnosis, care and treatment have emerged. Previously, physical and mental decline were assumed to be an inevitable consequence of the ageing process. Psychological needs are often forgotten. For example, quiet undemanding clients may not indicate the need for active care. However, this does not mean that such care is not required. An understanding of the potential problems will ensure positive mental health.

Changes such as cognition, mood, behaviour and personality are often the first indicators of a problem. They may be both subtle and complex and consequently demand precise and objective assessment. The best way of achieving this is by asking the older person. By telling their own story, in their own words they will often give prompts to the nurse who should be receptive to such cues. The skill of encouraging an open dialogue should be handled sensitively in an unhurried and unobtrusive manner, whilst maintaining privacy and confidentiality.

While, in the context of this chapter, it is impossible to address all the contributing factors that may predispose to mental illness in old age, care staff need to have an understanding of such basic issues as loss, bereavement, transition and loneliness. They also need to recognise that whilst the individual may not enter a care home with a mental illness it is possible to develop a mental health need through the effects of physical ill-health and/or environmental factors.

In this context it is worth noting that whilst some people may be able to articulate and describe the location of a physical problem, they are often unwilling or unable to describe such symptoms as feeling sad, or being 'down in the dumps'.

The social world to which an individual belongs (the context of their life before they came into the care home setting and the impact of it in their new surroundings), is an important predisposing factor to their mental health. A helpful method for assessing this is the use of biography. Life history will provide evidence of key elements in their past life which has brought them where they are today. Such milestones might include:

- childhood experiences,
- work,
- marriage,
- family relationships, and
- significant losses and relationships in life and how they have been adjusted to.

All of these will help the nurse form a better understanding of the individuals' behaviour within their care, recognising the individuals' right to choice and self-expression. There are rights relating to social participation too. It is not the simple choice of whether an individual participates or not, but how such social interaction relates to their own personality. Positive mental health will only be achieved by ensuring this balance reflects the individual's own interests and involvement. For example the man who has spent his life working alone and playing Bridge as a pastime may be horrified to have to join in the Saturday night bingo session.

Challenging behaviour

In working with people who have mental health needs, it is important to understand how to deal with 'abnormal' behaviour. The first thing to make clear is that there is no agreed definition of what is difficult or challenging. What would be considered by some as acceptable behaviour would cause others concern. To complicate matters even further people often have a model in their head of how old people should behave and these values are included in their mind-set. Imagine a man who is constantly trying to get out of his chair. Perhaps this seems unsafe, as a result he may be repeatedly put back into his chair and given no reason for this action. Yet he may wish to go to the toilet, to walk about, to look out of the window. His mental health problem may make it unlikely that he will accept the nurse's explanation as to why he should stay in the chair. His condition may affect his wish to constantly walk around.

Who has got the problem here: the client or the carer? The client is mentally ill, has problems in communication but the carer can also have a problem with a lack of imagination, sensitivity, gentleness or attention and perhaps different perceptions of the situation, and expectations of the older person to conform.

The important thing to remember is that the client is not the cause of the problem, but suffers the effects of the problem just as much, if not more so than the carer. It is also advisable to stand back and analyse the problem, rather than rushing in with a quick solution.

Kitwood and Bredin (1992) suggests considering the following:

- Is it really a problem and how often does it occur?
- Why is it a problem?
- Who is it a problem for? Have we, as caregivers, made it into a problem by being unwilling to change, adapt and accept?
- Is the person with the problem trying to tell us something
- How can this problem be resolved in a way which most enhances the persons' quality of life?

The care team should be aware of the client's assessment, mental health status, and act accordingly. Staff must recognise the right to express needs and wants, however this is demonstrated.

To make this work effectively it is important for care staff to use their skill in assessing the situation and interpreting their client's needs. Not only does this require a recognition of their needs, but some positive steps will have to be taken to alter the situation.

The more common types of behaviour experienced in care homes are: wandering, aggression, verbal communication, incontinence, sexually inappropriate behaviour and delusions/hallucinations.

Wandering

Trying to restrict wandering is probably the worst course of action here. Allowing the person to wander in a safe environment is a much better solution, as people have particular reasons for wandering, e.g. searching for a person, object or security. Not all wandering is related to confusion as many people think. Individuals should be allowed to express themselves, and to take risks in an environment which after all is their home. Opportunities need to be provided for them to have freedom and movement so that they can express themselves in ways that are meaningful and safe.

Aggression

The usual causes of aggression are responses to frustration and insecurity; for example, the person who is unable to communicate that they are in pain. It may be that they are also frustrated with their own powerlessness and find this the only way to express this frustration.

Verbal communication

The effects of mental illness or organic impairment may sometimes cause the older person to display certain types of behaviour that can be repetitive, causing annoyance to other residents and care staff. There are many possible reasons why the individual may repeat certain words, scream or make other noises and it is left to the skill of the carer to interpret the meanings behind these behaviours. It may be that the individual is extremely anxious, worried or has felt isolated for long periods of time (see Chapter 10).

Continence

As with all forms of incontinence, assessment is required. Sometimes incontinence can be the result of a physical problem such as a urinary tract infection or as a side effect of drug therapy. It may also be affected by immobility which restricts movement when attempting to visit the toilet. In some cases, however, incontinence may well result from damage that is occurring in the brain: the person can't remember where the toilet is, or recognise the signs that their bladder is full, or remember what the lavatory is for and may use other similar receptacles. It is important that the carer assesses each individual's need and devises an individually appropriate response (see Chapter 14).

Sexually inappropriate behaviour

Sexual relationships are of course a very private and personal matter, and a subject that many find uncomfortable or embarrassing to discuss. Whilst many mental health problems may not directly affect sexual relationships, the individual's attitude towards sexual activity may decline or alter. If partners are no longer recognised then other residents may be mistaken for partners and consequent attempts at sexual expression may take place. Staff need to be non-judgemental, understanding and skilled in such circumstances.

Sometimes a person with dementia may exhibit inappropriate behaviour, such as undressing in front of other residents, or fondling their genitals. This behaviour is unlikely to be sexual in nature but more to do with their cognitive impairment. It may be that they think it is time to get undressed, are totally unaware of their surroundings, or the presence of others, or are looking for the lavatory. Such behaviours can be embarrassing to carers and other residents, but should be managed calmly and the dignity maintained of all those concerned. Clues to the behaviour should be sought and responded to appropriately.

It is also important to remember that most people irrespective of age still have sexual needs and desires. Sexual feelings don't go away just because individual mental functioning declines. For some individuals, as parts of the brain functions reduce, the barriers that have previously inhibited them from acting on sexual desires are reduced. Expressing sexuality includes many aspects such as warmth and affection, having physical contact with others, the feelings of being accepted and a need to express one's own sexuality.

Carers can respond to most of these needs, but it is also important that we recognise and understand those clients who have the need to express their sexuality, and ensure that every individual is afforded the same privacy to be able to do so.

Delusions and hallucinations

A delusion can be defined as a suspicious idea that becomes a fixed belief, and one that cannot be eliminated by logical argument. For example an individual may believe that they are a member of the royal family when they are not. An hallucination on the other hand can be defined as a falsely recognised stimulus that can be both visual, auditory, tactile and olfactory. An example of this may be the belief that they have insects crawling over them. As can be imagined these experiences will be very frightening for the individual, but it is important not to collude with them. It is also worth noting that older people have a tendency to develop both visual and hearing deficiencies, so any evidence of genuine physical causes should be investigated and eliminated first.

Other behaviours

In all situations which produce challenging behaviours, the carer should focus on the person rather than the problem behaviour.

Although not always seen as a challenging behaviour, complaints can cause difficulty and perhaps the labelling of an individual as a trouble maker. It is important to remember that just because the client does not articulate their complaint in what is accepted as the normal way, does not mean that their complaint is not valid.

For example people may refuse to eat for a variety of reasons. It may be for a religious or cultural reason, or it may simply be because they do not like the food. The world is full of people, of all ages, who do not like some foods, who complain about its quality, and who have their own preferences and routines. Moves towards customer care in this country mean that organisations such as restaurants go out of their way to ensure these complaints are dealt with. What is the difference in a care home? Why should the client not be offered choice, or the opportunity to question openly without fear of reprisal?

There may be complaints about other clients with whom they share a room. Maybe they snore; maybe that person is used to having a room of their own and certainly not sharing it with someone who they never met until they entered the home. Of course everyone has rights to the treatment they receive, and communal living is bound to cause some disagreement and compromise, but the key issue is that the their complaints can be valid. Very few people are difficult or display anti-social behaviour all of the time, but if they are labelled in those terms, the positive elements of their personalities are often ignored.

In all cases of challenging behaviour the carer should try to find a detailed explanation for the way the client is behaving by familiarising themselves with life history and patterns of behaviour. Every problem must be individually assessed. The carer will need to ask themselves the following questions:

● What actually happens?
● When does it occur? (what are its antecedents?)
● Where does it happen?
● Who is it a problem for?

The carer needs to ensure that there is a consistent approach in managing behaviour by sharing information with colleagues and agreeing a uniform method of response. The principle is that the client's independence must be encouraged and respected and that any element of risk should be in the clients' favour whilst always looking for ways to minimise risk. The carer also needs to be aware of how their own attitudes can affect the way in which they respond to certain situations, and clients, whatever the degree of disability, will pick up these feelings, and respond accordingly.

It perhaps needs to be restated that the residents are not there to meet the criteria of the smooth running of the home's administration procedures, but rather that the home is there to meet the residents' varying needs be they mental, physical, psychological or social.

Guidelines for good practice

Whatever the area of care for older people, the principle of good practice needs to be paramount. It is therefore essential that everyone concerned with the care of older people is accountable for the quality nursing care which they provide. Essential to this process is the development of standards which provide a benchmark against which services are assessed.

In drawing up a set of standards the following principles need to be considered:

● The service should reflect the needs of the individual.
● The individual's right to privacy, independence, confidentiality and dignity should be maintained at all times.
● Older people and their advocates should be involved in, and make informed choices about their treatment and care.
● There should be clear, identifiable standards, which are specific enough to be easily put into practice.
● The standards should respond to the changing needs in both nursing practice and older people themselves.
● Older people should be valued and their worth recognised.

Conclusion

Nurses working with older people who have mental health needs may sometimes find it difficult to see the positive results of their efforts. It is easy to say that clients' needs are paramount but in practice such ideals may be difficult to meet day by day. Working with older people with mental health problems can be difficult. Unlike many other areas of nursing, the clients do not change very much over time.

Positive improvements may be small and not always easy to recognise, they need to be looked for carefully. It may be difficult for staff to see the impact of their work, and consequently they do not feel reward or satisfaction. As a result staff can often become de-skilled and demotivated if they have no support structures to help them. In the hospital and the community, clinical supervision, for example, is available to ensure the nurse recognises the broader context in which they are working and are less isolated in their situation. There is no reason why such a system could not be employed in a residential care home and this is covered more fully in Chapter 8. Finally, the need for expert and skilled nursing and medical involvement should not be underestimated. The Royal College of Nursing guidelines on mental health assessment (1993) do, however, assist the nurse who is not a registered mental health nurse, to recognise the principles of good practice and when to refer the client for expert assessment.

The key to effective care for older people with mental health needs is the recognition of the need for individualised treatment for the client. Myths around ill-health being synonymous with old age and what is considered age-appropriate behaviour are common and misleading. The only way to combat these is a genuine desire to know more about the individual through a sensitive and responsive professional relationship.

References

Alzeimer's Disease Society (1994) Alzheimer's Disease – What is it? Information sheet No. 1. Alzheimer's Disease Society.

Arie, T. (1981) *Health care of the elderly*. Croom Helm.

Bromley, D.B. (1978) Approaches to the study of personality changes in adult life and old age. In Isaacs, A.D. and Post F(eds) *Studies in Geriatric Psychiatry*, pp. 17–40. Chichester: Wiley.

Butterworth, C.A. and Faugier J. (1992) *Clinical Supervision and Mentorship in Nursing*. Chapman and Hall.

Capewell, A.R.E., Primrose, W.R. and MacIntyre, C. (1986) Nursing dependency in registered nursing homes and long-term geriatric wards in Edinburgh. *British Medical Journal*, 292, 1719–1721.

Davidson, K.M., Donoghue, I., Jackoby, R. et al. (1994) *Impact of Depression: A Multi-Disciplinary Comment on Treating Depression*. Lundbeck.

Davies, Wilkinson, S.J., Downes, J.T. et al. (1988) Global ratings of stress in the elderly. *British Journal of Clinical Psychology*, 27, 179–180.

Department of Health (1994) Mental illness: mental health and older people. HMSO.

Gidley, I and Shears, R. (1988) *Alzheimer's: What it is, How to Cope*. Unwin.

Hunt, A. (1979) Some aspects of the health of elderly people in England. *Health Trends*, 11, 21–23.

Kay, D.W.K. Beamish, T., Roth, M. (1964) Old age mental disorders in Newcastle-upon-Tyne Part 1: a study of prevalence. *British Journal of Psychiatry*, 110, 146–158.

Kellner, R. and Sheffield, B.E. (1973) A self-rating scale of distress. *Psychological Medicine*, 3, 88–100.

Kitwood, T. and Bredin, K. (1992) *Person to Person*. Gale Centre Publications.

Lindesay, J., Briggs, K., and Murphy, E. (1989). The Guy's/Age Concern Survey. Prevalence rates of cognitive impairment, depression and anxiety in an urban elderly community. *British Journal of Psychiatry*, 155, 317–329.

Murphy, E. (1992) Affective disorders in old age. In E.S. Paykel (ed.) *Handbook of Affective Disorders*. Churchill Livingstone.

Pearce, J. and Miller, E. (1973) *Clinical Aspects of Dementia*. Bailliere Tindall.

Ray, J.J. (1988) Lie scales and the elderly. *Personality and Individual Differences*, **4**, 17-22.

Royal College of Nursing (1993) Guidelines for assessing mental health needs in old age. Royal College of Nursing.

Royal College of Physicians/British Geriatrics Society (1992) High quality long-term care for elderly people: Guidelines and audit measures. Royal College of Physicians.

Sim, M., Turner, E., Smith, W.T. (1966) Cerebral biopsy in the investigation of pre-senile dementia. *British Journal of Psychiatry*, **112**, 119–125.

Sjogren, T, Sjogren, H. and Lindgren, A.G.H. (1952) Morbus Alzheimer and morbus Pick: a genetic, clinical and pathoanatomical study. *Acta Psychiatrica et Neurologica Scandinavica*, **82**, 1–152.

UKCC (1994) Professional conduct – occasional report on standards of nursing in nursing homes. United Kingdom Central Council for Nursing, Midwifery and Health Visiting.

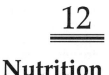

12

Nutrition

Andrée LeMay

Introduction

Eating and drinking are central elements in all our lives, not only from the perspective of maintaining our health but also as a means of socialising with friends and relatives, and for cultural or religious reasons. During a lifetime each of us develops likes and dislikes, favourite foods and foods and drinks which we would choose above others.

Alongside this we each develop preferences about the atmosphere in which we eat and drink: in company, alone, in front of the television or reading a newspaper. All of these experiences and preferences will affect the way an older person, living in a care home, considers nutrition. Nutrition is a central issue in the continuing care of older people living in care homes. Not only does nutritional status impact on physical health, but it also influences psychological and social well-being. In this chapter I intend to bring these issues together, with the aim of encouraging a nutritional awareness which meets individual needs.

Admission to a care home can cause disruptions to a person's usual diet, times and frequently of meals, and the social aspects related to eating (Chenitz, Stone and Salisbury, 1991). These may be compounded by diminished health, feelings of isolation, previous neglect, and underlying signs of malnourishment.

Denham (1992) emphasises the importance of nutritional status for the older person when he writes:

> An unbalanced diet in later life, caused by either too much food, or a specific deficiency, may shorten life expectancy or increase morbidity due to age-related diseases. A carefully planned and balanced diet, however, especially if combined with regular exercise, is likely to maintain health, improve life expectancy and quality of life.

This, of course, is equally true for any older person wherever they live.

For anyone living in a care home food may be a highlight of the day. It is therefore important that food is appetising, nutritionally appropriate, and served attractively in convivial surroundings with appropriate utensils and equipment and tables and chairs of a correct height (Fenton, 1989). Seen together these points emphasise the physical, social and psychological importance of food and eating.

Nurses have many roles in relation to nutrition, from assessment and monitoring through to involvement in the planning of menus and meal times. Although this role is not isolated from other members of the multi-disciplinary team, the nurse is likely, through continued knowledge of the older client, to be the first to observe changes in nutritional status.

Some basic facts about nutrition

Nutrients are 'Chemical constituents of food necessary for proper body functioning: to supply us with energy, aid in the growth and repair of body tissues and help in the regulation of body processes.' (Kart, Metress and Metress, 1992); and can be categorised as carbohydrates, fats, proteins, minerals and vitamins. Water and flavours/colours should be added to this list as they are also constituents of foods (Ministry of Agriculture, Fisheries and Food, 1993).

Carbohydrates provide the body with energy and may be converted into body fat (MAFF, 1993). The three main groups are sugars, starches and non-starch polysaccharides (dietary fibre). Dietary sugars (e.g. glucose, fructose and sucrose) provide between 10 and 20 per cent of food energy (DoH, 1992). Links between certain sugars and dental caries are well known and therefore reductions should be aimed for in relation to high sugar-content foods/drinks (confectionary, soft drinks) to ensure older people keep their teeth for as long as possible. These sugars also contain 'empty' energy and as such may blunt people's appetites for other foods (DoH, 1992).

The Department of Health (1992) recommend that older adults increase their intake of starchy foods such as bread and potatoes and the Nutrition Advisory Group for the Elderly (NAGE) in 1992 suggested at least one portion from this nutrient group should be eaten daily (see Table 12.1). In the case of non-starch polysaccharides (NSP), their importance in preventing constipation is emphasised and an intake of 12–18 grams per day is recommended (DoH, 1992). NSP are found in wholegrain cereals, pulses and some vegetables and fruit. Many older people already enjoy these foods but for those with chewing difficulties care will be need to be taken in their preparation.

Fats also provide energy and again, may be converted into body fat (MAFF, 1993). Kart, Metress and Metress (1992) remind us that fat should be limited to less than 25–30 per cent of total energy intake due to the links drawn between fat consumption and cardio-vascular disease. However, care does need to be taken to ensure that fat consumption is not reduced to such an extent as to compromise the absorption of fat-soluble vitamins (A, D, E and K), and to make the diet unpalatable and monotonous.

Proteins provide materials (amino acids) for growth and repair. They can also be converted into carbohydrate and therefore become a source of energy (MAFF, 1993). The UK Reference Nutrient Intakes for protein for people aged over 50 are 46.5 grams per day (women) and 53.3 grams per day (men) (DoH, 1991). However, a year later the Department of Health (1992) suggested that further research was needed to determine precisely the protein requirements of older people. NAGE (1992) provided daily targets for protein rich foods (Table 12.1).

Vitamins help to regulate the body processes (MAFF, 1993) and can be divided into those which are fat soluble (A, D, E and K) and those which are water soluble (C and B complex).

Minerals are used for growth and repair and help to regulate body processes (MAFF, 1993).

Table 12.1   *Daily nutritional targets (adapted from NAGE, 1992)*

	Provision for each resident
Milk (full cream)	Half to one pint daily
Meat	2/3 oz portion when cooked
Fish	4/5 oz portion when cooked
Pulses	4 oz portion when cooked
Cheese	2 oz portion when cooked
Eggs	
	Select 2 portions from list
Bread	Provide 1 or more helping
Breakfast cereals	of one of these at each meal
Pasta	
Rice	Portion size will vary with
Potatoes	appetite
Vegetables (fresh/frozen)	At least 2 portions daily
Salad	
Fruit (fresh/dried/stewed/tinned)	Include one portion daily
Fruit juice	
Fluids	At least 8 cups daily

The Department of Health (1992) issued updated information regarding the nutrition of elderly people based on earlier work (DoH, 1991) on dietary reference values for good energy and nutrients for people aged over 50 in the United Kingdom. You may find it useful to consult these tables but should bear in mind that these relate to healthy people living independently. Residents in nursing homes may have specific needs which you might wish to discuss with a dietitian.

Additionally residents will have personal preferences, likes and dislikes, and should be fully involved in decisions affecting them.

NAGE (1992) provides some useful nutritional targets which directly relate to various types of food and drink. I think these would be a sound starting point and have therefore summarised them in Table 12.1

Special considerations for older people

Several writers state that there is no evidence to suggest that nutrient requirements diminish with age (Kart, Metress and Metress, 1992; NAGE, 1992). However, there is agreement that energy requirements are generally reduced. This reduction is associated with diminished physical activity and a decline in basal metabolic rate (DoH, 1991). The reduction, however, may result in limited variety in the diet so special attention is needed to ensure that foods contain sufficient protein, vitamins, minerals and trace elements to maintain a balanced diet.

The Department of Health (1991) suggested estimated average daily requirements for energy (according to weight, sex and age) as being:

For men
65–74 years   71 kg   2330 kal per day
75+ years   69 kg   2100 kcal per day

For women
65–74 years   63 kg   1900 kcal per day
75+ years   60 kg   1810 kcal per day

Take care, however, to ensure that individual health status and weight are taken into account when determining energy requirements. This is an ideal starting point for professional collaboration and seeking expert advice from dietitians.

Holmes (1994) summarises age-related changes which may affect the older person's nutritional requirements. These include:

● diminished senses of smell, taste, touch and sight;
● reduced secretion of saliva which may make chewing and swallowing more difficult than in the past;
● gastrointestinal changes (for example: loss of teeth, decreased hydrochloric acid secretion with resultant reduction in the absorption of calcium and iron;
● oesophageal changes resulting in dysphagia, heartburn and epigastric discomfort and reduced mobility in the gastrointestinal tract (often culminating in constipation);
● poor dentition, ranging from loss of teeth to inefficient chewing to ill fitting dentures which make eating painful;
● altered metabolism centring on reduced basal metabolic rate and diminished glucose tolerance; and
● reduced renal function which leads to the inefficient handling of waste produces and/or electrolytes.

Together with these age-related changes, there are specific health issues which may affect older people and indeed may have led to their admission to a nursing home. It is worth considering these individually.

Dysphagia

Swallowing difficulties can occur for a number of different reasons (e.g. stroke, Parkinson's disease, cancer). Whatever their cause, they can significantly affect the nutritional status of the individual because of reduced nutrient intake (Damon, 1988). Andrews (1987) suggests simple measures to reduce these problems, such as finding an easily swallowed type of food and ensuring an erect posture when sitting down to eat.

Musculoskeletal and neurological disorders

Arthritis, paralysis, impaired vision and aphasia (loss of speech) may all interfere with nutritional status through either direct physical disability or inability to state food preferences.

Poor dental health

This encompasses both dental and periodontal disease which may culminate in the loss of teeth. This can lead to problems related to food consumption as chewing becomes difficult, resulting in a limited diet composed of soft foods, which lack texture and variety. These foods may also be low in fibre and unappetisingly monotonous. Fenton (1989) reminds us that soft mince, frequently used as the base of a soft diet, may resemble a lumpy soup which is itself a poor texture for anyone whose poor dental health is compounded by swallowing difficulties. This illustrates the need for a complete nutritional assessment since many residents may have more than one nutritional problem.

Dementia

Older people with dementia are likely to have nutritional problems related to altered eating patterns. Watson (1994a) reviewed the literature in relation to the range of problems which may be experienced: dysphagia, refusal to eat, diminished ability to feed oneself, problems keeping food in the mouth, and spitting. I have found his articles (Watson, 1993; 1994a,b; Watson and Deary, 1994) useful in putting together a comprehensive picture which can help nurses to identify challenges related to dementia and nutrition whilst suggesting some basic interventions. Watson's work emphasises the need to assess residents individually to determine the level of difficulty that they experience, assessing refusal to eat, spitting and dysphagia. This assessment can then indicate individual interventions and care can be planned and evaluated appropriately.

NAGE (1992) also offers some useful pointers for consideration. Ensure close supervision of meals and observe for choking, dehydration and poor communication. Identify with each resident their own place at the dining table to encourage a sense of 'belonging' and prompt residents to eat when they forget. Never force a person to eat, and offer a meal alternative (e.g. milk and sandwiches) if food is refused. Encourage careful menu planning coupled with individual plans related to nutritional care for each resident, considering energy requirements and nutrient intakes.

Depression

Holmes (1994) draws attention to the nutritional consequences of depression. Frequently characterised by erratic eating patterns with some people eating very little and others eating more than usual. Either may lead to malnutrition.

Dehydration

Many older people are vulnerable to dehydration because of the combination of a diminished ability to concentrate urine and fluid restriction. The latter may frequently be associated with attempts to control urinary incontinence (Kennedy, 1988). The link between dehydration and confusion in some old people is well known, and is in fact a double edged sword as the potential for confusion may hinder adequate food intake too.

Stroke

Eating and drinking problems commonly accompany strokes. Several are noted in the literature but I have chosen to focus on three: lip function, food pocketing and positioning. Carr and Hawthorn (1988) investigated lip function and eating in people following a stroke. They found that although food often collected around the lips of stroke patients, they were slow to clear it away, despite being aware of it. This may be because of poor muscle tone in the lips, weakness of muscles related to mouth opening, poor tongue function or poor lip seal. These problems may be worsened by reduced manual control or visuospatial problems. They suggested that nurses could try to increase a person's awareness by showing or describing what is happening during eating and encouraging them to do oral exercises.

A reduction in these difficulties may lessen embarrassment, increase nutritional intake and make eating and drinking more enjoyable experiences. This study really indicates the strong link between the physical, psychological and social elements of nutrition, and highlights how nurses can increase their role in rehabilitation and nutritional care to promote general well-being.

Some people who have had a stroke unintentionally pocket food in their mouths after meals. The nurse must be aware of this and check if necessary. Some will be able to use their tongue to locate the remaining food and then spit it out, whilst others will need the nurse to manually remove the food. Failure to ensure that the mouth is clear may cause later aspiration of the unswallowed food.

Finally, appropriate positioning during meals is of central importance to someone who has had a stroke and has resultant swallowing difficulties. Thomas (1991) states:

> Wherever possible the (older person) should sit in a chair, rather than in bed. Feet should be flat on the floor, ensuring good flexion of the hips. In the case of the stroke patient, the affected side of the body should be brought forward, by lifting the weaker arm onto the table.

Whilst this list is not exhaustive it provides an understanding of the complexity of nutrition in later life when age-related changes are compounded by chronic illness. It is important, though, to remember that acute illness (for example, the presence of pressure sores, fractures or infections) also affects nutritional status and specialist advice should be sought in relation to specific nutritional needs associated with these.

Frequently older people are taking medications which themselves influence nutritional status. Kart, Metress and Metress (1992) suggested two links between drugs and nutrition. The first is that drugs affect nutrient absorption and metabolism, and the second that nutritional and health status may affect drug metabolism.

Malnourishment in older people

In 1990 Swedish researchers reported that 28.5 per cent of patients, in their study of 482 elderly people, suffered from protein-energy malnutrition shortly after admission for long-term care (Larsson, Unosson, Ek et al., 1990). However, the potential for malnourishment does not stop at admission to a long-term care facility. This has been emphasised by Peggy Yen (1989) in an American survey which found that 85 per cent of elderly people living in nursing homes and hospitals were malnourished.

Chenitz, Stone and Salisbury (1991) identified factors which may lead to what they term iatrogenic malnutrition; these include illness-related factors (polypharmacy, pain, reduced mobility, loss of appetite, dietary restriction and poorly fitting dentures) and institution-related factors. Both are important for you to consider but the institution-related factors may be particularly so, as in many instances they will be within your control (Table 12.2)

Davies and Holdsworth (1979) studied the nutritional status of older people living in residential homes and identified several risk factors which may predispose a person to malnourishment: monotonous diet, the last meal by 5 pm each day, limited choice, low fibre content and a lack of knowledge regarding nutrients by those preparing meals. This sort of information is useful to have as it highlights where practice can be improved as well as emphasising the importance of nutrition in the everyday care of an older adult requiring continuing care. Nutritional status has far-reaching consequences and as such is a vital element of skilled nursing practice. The factors identified should be borne in mind as you read the next section of this chapter.

Table 12.2:   *Institutional issues which may promote malnutrition (Chenitz, Stone and Salisbury, 1991)*

- Unmet cultural/personal dietary preferences;
- changed meal times;
- unfamiliar eating partners;
- inappropriate and difficult packaging;
- unpleasant environment in which to eat;
- lack of oral care;
- lack of handwashing;
- lack of dentures, glasses or hearing aids;
- use of restraint; and
- scheduling procedures to co-ordinate with mealtimes.

Ensuring good nutrition in the home

Nurses have a central function in ensuring good standards of nutritional care for everyone living in a nursing home. Currently both the Royal College of Nursing (1993) and the Nutritional Advisory Group for the Elderly (1992) provide valuable advise related to nutrition in later life. Both publications emphasise the provision of high standards of nutritional care. The Royal College of Nursing (1993) has produced a national set of guidelines called 'Nutrition Standards and the Older Adult'. These are presented as a series of standards which aim to help nurses to 'improve the nutritional care and consequent nutritional status of older adults in continuing care'. Three standards form the basis of this document:

1. Assessment of past and/or potential difficulties in eating and drinking.
2. Enabling the client to eat and drink.
3. Monitoring and evaluating the nutritional status and nutritional care of the clients.

Within each, emphasis is placed on specific issues which should form a template for care. Assessment focuses on the initial assessment of the client's nutritional status and involves asking the client and his or her relatives about food and fluid intake and eating habits. By contrast, 'enabling the client to eat and drink' emphasises the multi-disciplinary nature of facilitating eating and drinking by reminding the nurse to meet regularly with catering managers, dietitians and speech therapists, and other members of the multi-disciplinary team. The standard emphasises a client-centred approach, where choice over menu content and the timing of meals is encouraged, with meals being served in a 'pleasurable ambience'. Documentation of nutritional care is advocated and this, in turn, affects the third standard. This final standard relates to the monitoring and evaluation of care and emphasises the need for nurses to maintain their involvement in order to determine changes to a client's food and drink preferences and their ability to maintain a satisfactory nutritional status.

NAGE (1992) complements the Royal College of Nursing (1993) standards by providing specific information related to nutritional targets for older people, ideas for meals (including vegetarian meals, soft diets and liquidised meals), menu planning and the timing of meals, religious food preferences and advice regarding the use of supplements. Therapeutic diets are considered (diabetic, weight control, low fat, high protein) as well as the role of fibre. This handbook is specifically designed for those involved in providing meals for older people and may be a useful starting place for bringing all those concerned with the nutritional culture of the home together. To help to link these ideas it may be useful to have an individual checklist which acts as an aide memoire when focusing on each resident. This checklist (Figure 12.1) will help you to

---

Nutritional checklist

■ Assessment   (date......................)

■ Menu planning:...
■ Meal times:..
■ Situation of meals: ....
■ Special requests:..
■ Special equipment/extra support from nurse:...............................
....

■ Liaison with other specialists:...
■ Referral to other specialists: ....
....

■ Frequency of monitoring:...
■ Evaluation of nutritional plan: ....
....

■ Choice emphasised:...
....
....

Resident............................ Nurse..............................

Figure 12.1   *Nutritional Checklist*

gain information from each resident and can be used in conjunction with the assessment procedures described later in this chapter, whilst also reminding you of information to pass on to the resident in relation to eating and drinking in the home.

The principles of good nutrition centre on the provision of a nutritionally balanced diet which allows residents choice over food and drink. This is delivered in an appetising and pleasant way which encourages people to enjoy their food in a convivial environment and promotes social interaction.

Residents who need extra support with eating and drinking should receive the help necessary to enhance and maintain their nutritional status. All residents should have a nutritional assessment when they are admitted and this should be regularly reviewed through individual evaluation and monitoring.

Nutritional assessment

Assessment is an essential component of nutritional care since without it a sensitive nutritional plan cannot be formulated and monitored. The literature abounds with various recommendations related to assessment techniques including anthropometric (body weight, height, skinfold thickness and limb muscle circumferences and areas) (Goodinson, 1987), and biochemical assessment (Collingsworth, 1991). It is not my intention to discuss these two further but to focus on information which will enable you to develop a greater understanding of each resident's nutritional status through history taking and observation. By doing this it is anticipated that you will be able to identify those at risk of malnourishment, gain knowledge of each resident's food preferences and monitor nutritional care on an individual and institutional basis.

Thomas (1991) provides useful starting points for assessment through history taking. These start by finding out:

● diagnosis/reason for admission,
● drug therapy,
● weight,
● social history,
● dietary history,
● number of meals per day,
● content of meals,
● timing of meals,
● consumption of alcohol, and
● daily fluid consumption.

However, Denham (1992) advises care in relation to obtaining this sort of historical information since, he suggests that dietary histories are subject to vagaries of human memory so you may find it helpful to supplement this information by asking relatives and carers as well as residents.

Nottingham City Hospital NHS Trust (1993) have devised a nutritional assessment chart which focuses on diet, swallowing, ability to feed oneself, mouth condition and the condition of the skin. This chart includes a scoring system which suggests that a score of 14 or below denotes nutritional risk necessitating referal to a dietitian. This type of scale is easy to use and can be used over a period of time to determine change in relation to nutritional risk. You can find a copy of this scale in the Royal College of Nursing (1993) nutritional standards booklet.

Observing meals may also provide supplementary information related to each resident's eating behaviours. It may be possible to determine difficulties experienced with utensils, the amount and type of food eaten, the length of time taken to eat a meal and the social interaction which occurs during the meal. All of this information is useful in developing knowledge about each resident's nutritional requirements.

Good nursing

Appropriate nursing care centres on enabling the client to receive a nutritionally balanced diet. This involves, on an individual resident basis, ensuring that a plan of care is devised which focuses on setting nutritional goals, collaboratively with residents and other professionals. This focuses on negotiation and choice, so that each older person feels able to choose their favourite dishes and drinks from time to time, as well as choosing meals from a routinely available selection. Once this is achieved several general principles related to good nursing practices should be attended to.

Mouth and denture care are of great importance. Dentures should be labelled to guard against misuse and care should be taken to check that they fit correctly and are not uncomfortable. For those who do not have dentures, oral care is equally important and some residents may need help to maintain adequate levels of oral hygiene. Referral for regular dental checks continues to be important in later life (Wright, 1988) and Thomas (1991) suggests that dentures should be replaced every five to ten years. In some instances specific diseases or treatments may affect oral health and care needs to be taken to ensure the highest possible standards. Good oral care may need to be coupled with dietary changes to ensure adequate nutritional status and once again advice from a dietitian should be sought.

Reducing the risk of constipation can be achieved by encouraging residents to eat fibre-containing foods such as wholemeal bread, wholegrain cereals (Weetabix, Porridge Oats, and All Bran), peas, beans, lentils, and carrots, pears and apples with their skins on (NAGE, 1992). These foods should be coupled with an adequate fluid intake (at least eight cups each day) since fibre absorbs water (NAGE, 1992).

Exercise is another important consideration and has been mentioned earlier in relation to energy requirements. For some residents this may mean walking in the garden or going to local parks or shops. Others may enjoy taking part in indoor fitness groups which focus on gentle exercise, or music and movement classes. Exercise may lessen the likelihood of constipation, stimulate the appetite and enhance feelings of psychological and social well-being.

Appropriate feeding and drinking aids and equipment should be selected by the nurse to suit each individual resident's requirements. Wright (1988) emphasis the importance of ensuring that the client is sitting comfortably in an upright position with normal utensils and equipment (chair and table) whenever possible. When special aids and equipment are needed, such as non-slip mats or adapted cutlery, it is essential that they are used appropriately and that independence is maximised. Thomas (1991) draws attention to the demoralisation that may be associated with using a feeding cup and suggests that whenever possible cups and glasses should be used with straws. Together with these points, a relaxed, attractive atmosphere should be created by considering tableware, flowers and lighting. These may greatly increase residents' enjoyment of eating and drinking. Inclusion of residents in these decisions will also enhance their feeling of control and self-esteem.

In line with this, Damon (1988) discusses the importance of proper positioning in relation to feeding clients. She stresses the unsuitability of feeding someone who is in a recumbent position with their necks hyper-extended since this position makes swallowing difficult and increases the risk of aspiration into the tracheobronchial tree.

Providing appropriate food

There is much debate about which foods and drinks are healthy. Many older people will have differing views to those currently accepted and these will have influenced the way in which their dietary patterns have developed. Over-zealous attention to a nutritionally balanced, healthy diet which cuts out all the foods or drinks which that person has found appetising and enjoyable may cause great distress to them. A balance between the two approaches is a hallmark of good care.

NAGE (1992) provides a useful summary of some religious food preferences which are displayed in Table 12.3. Special preparation requirements are also necessary for Muslims and Orthodox Jews and many religions include an element of fasting which may be important to your residents.

Table 12.3:   *Religious food preferences (adapted from NAGE, 1992)*

Foods/drinks	Acceptable	Not acceptable
Eggs	Most Muslims Some Sikhs	Strict Hindus and Sikhs
Milk, yoghurt, butter/ghee	Muslims, Sikhs and Hindus	
Cheese	Some Muslims, Sikhs and Hindus	
Mutton	Halal for Muslims Some Sikhs and Hindus	Strict Hindus and Sikhs
Beef	Halal for Muslims	All Sikhs and Hindus

It is also important to remember special requirements related to the three types of vegetarian diets (lacto-vegetarian, lacto-ovo-vegetarian and vegan) and to seek advice regarding the nutritional content of these in relation to each individual resident. The basic principles of these diets are highlighted in Table 12.4.

Table 12.4:   *Components of vegetarian diets (Nage, 1992)*

Lacto-vegetarians	Eat milk and dairy products
	Do not eat eggs, meat, poultry, or fish
Lacto-ovo-vegetarians	Eat milk, dairy products and eggs
	Do not eat meat, poultry, or fish
Vegans	Eat vegetables, fruit and cereals
	Do not eat any animal products

Whilst considering the provision of appropriate foods it is also necessary to consider how foods are provided. Some people have particular habits which affect their enjoyment of food, for instance where they eat their food, (sitting at a table, sitting in front of the television), the use of particular utensils (e.g. napkins) or the way a table is laid for a meal. All of these may impinge on the nutritional status of people and can make a difference to the nutritional culture in which they live.

Eating and drinking are social occasions and have particular importance when associated with feelings of celebration or commiseration (e.g. birthdays, funerals, religious events). Elderly residents may welcome the opportunity to keep these rituals especially as they may be isolated from close family and friends who may, in the past, have been central to these events. Special foods may also help to maintain feelings of well-being and bring back fond memories (for example, fish and chips from a fish and chip shop) as may trips to local pubs or restaurants. Nurses who are sensitive to cultural, religious and ethnic groups' specific likes and needs will strive to ensure that individual needs can be met in the community of the home.

Many people experience feelings of fulfilment and creativity through the preparation of foods and drinks, and wherever possible this should be encouraged. Ideas to facilitate this range from groups of residents preparing dishes for others to arranging social functions which involve eating and drinking. This involvement may increase feelings of self-esteem and promote well-being.

Conclusion

The relationship between physical, psychological and social well-being is central to nutritional care within a care home, being intrinsically linked to each resident's enjoyment of eating and drinking. This chapter emphasises the central role of the nurse in providing individualised care to help residents to plan their diet, the timing of their meals, and then monitor their nutritional intake. This all-round approach is likely to highlight nutritional problems, issues related to wastage, and to help identify malnourishment at an earlier stage than if the nurse did not take on this responsibility.

References

Andrews, K. (1987) *Rehabilitation of the Older Adult.* Edward Arnold.

Carr, E. and Hawthorne, P. (1988) Lip function and eating after a stroke: A nursing perspective. *Journal of Advanced Nursing,* **13,** 447–451.

Chenitz, W., Stone, J. and Salisbury, S. (1991) *Clinical Gerontological Nursing.* W B Saunders.

Collingsworth, R. (1991) Determining nutritional status of the elderly surgical patient: Steps in the assessment process. *AORN Journal,* **54,** 3, 622–631.

Damon, J. (1988) Nutritional considerations. In: M. Matteson and E. McConnell (eds) *Gerontological Nursing: Concepts and Practice.* W B Saunders.

Davies, L. and Holdsworth, M. (1979) A Technique for Assessing Nutritional 'at risk' Factors in Residential Homes for the Elderly. *Journal of Human Nutrition,* **33,** 165–169.

Denham, M. (1992) Some Food for Thought. *Care of the Elderly,* October, 373–374.

Department of Health (1991) *Dietary Reference Values for Food Energy and Nutrients for the United Kingdom.* HMSO.

Department of Health (1992) *The Nutrition of Elderly People.* HMSO.

Fenton, J. (1989) Some food for thought. *Health Services Journal,* 1st June, 666–667.

Goodinson, S. (1987) Anthropometric assessment of nutritional status. *Professional Nurse,* September, 388–393.

Holmes, S. (1994) Nutrition and older people: a matter of concern. *Nursing Times,* **90,** 42, 31–33.

Kart, C., Metress, E. and Metress, S. (1992) *Human Aging and Chronic Disease.* Jones and Bartlett Publishers.

Kennedy, A. (1988) *Eliminating.* In S. Wright (ed.) *Nursing the Older Patient.* Lippincott.

Larsson, J., Unosson, M., Ek, A. et al. (1990) Effect of dietary supplement on nutritional status and clinical outcome in 501 geriatric patients: a randomised study. *Clinical Nutrition,* **9,** 179–184.

Ministry of Agriculture, Fisheries and Food (1993) *Manual of Nutrition.* London: HMSO.

NAGE (1990) Nutrition Assessment Checklist. Nutrition Advisory Group for the Elderly.

NAGE (1992) Eating through the 90s. Nutrition Advisory Group for the Elderly.

Nottingham City Hospital NHS Trust (1993) Nutritional Assessment Chart. In Royal College of Nursing (1993) *Nutritional Standards and the Older Adult*. RCN.

Royal College of Nursing (1993) Nutrition Standards and the Older Adult. RCN.

Thomas, S. (1991) Eating and Drinking. In S. Redfern (ed.) *Nursing Elderly People*. Churchill Livingstone.

Watson, R. (1993) Measuring feeding difficulty in patients with dementia: perspectives and problems. *Journal of Advanced Nursing*, **18**, 25–31.

Watson, R. (1994a) Measuring feeding difficulty in patients with dementia: developing a scale. *Journal of Advanced Nursing*, **19**, 257–263.

Watson (1994b) Measuring feeding difficulty in patients with dementia: replication and validation of the EdFED Scale #1. *Journal of Advanced Nursing*, **19**, 850–855.

Watson, R. and Deary, I. (1994) Measuring feeding difficulty in patients with dementia: multivariate analysis of feeding problems, nursing intervention and indicators of feeding difficulty. *Journal of Advanced Nursing*, **20**, 283–287.

Wright, S. (1988) Eating and Drinking. In S. Wright (ed.) *Nursing the Older Patient*. Lippincott.

Yen, P. (1989) The Picture of Malnutrition. *Geriatric Nursing*, May/June, 159.

Mobility

Jane Slack and Lynne Phair

Introduction

For older people living in care homes mobility difficulties are common. This is often a factor that has contributed to their inability to live independently. Yet, even for the more able-bodied older person, living at home, difficulties with walking outside, getting public transport, standing to do the cooking and cleaning; or washing and dressing can increasingly cause problems (Farquhar, Grundy and Formby, 1993). Natural exercise taken while performing household tasks is lost as peoples' mobility deteriorates and this in turn affects independence. Mobility is fundamental to a person's belief in him or herself as as independent person, and to lose mobility and movement can, for some, be a loss that is hard to bear.

The term mobility describes a range of activities. Examples include getting in or out of bed, getting out of a chair, sitting down or walking about. An older person's reactions and responses can be slowed either by the natural ageing process, or by a health need. It is important that the interrelationships of these are acknowledged by nurses and demonstrated through patience, understanding and empathy.

Assessment

Knowledge of both theory and practice must be incorporated by the nurse into a caring and understanding plan of care, which will have a direct impact on a person's movement and ability.

In order that the nurse may effectively assist and promote independent mobility with an older person, they must firstly assess how the individual is able to carry out activities associated with daily living.

In order for a nursing care plan to be successfully implemented, the nurse must have an in-depth knowledge of the ageing process and the various disease processes that can affect older people. The nurse should ascertain the abilities of the older person by both asking questions and observing the individual. Some of the points that the nurse should observe in assessment are:

● How does the person stand? Are they off balance?
● When walking what is their gait, is if shuffling, is the foot being lifted off the floor adequately?

- Is the walking speed slower than normal, does it become slower the further the person walks?
- Are they able to transfer from bed to chair; is there difficulty in sitting or standing?
- Is the person unsteady when standing, does he/she try to catch hold of furniture in order to steady themselves?

The use of such assessment tools as the Barthel Index of Activities of Daily Living (ADL) (Kane and Kane, 1988) is good practice for all nurses assessing the functional ability of older people, and is particularly relevant to those working in a care home setting, where ongoing assessment is required.

The effects of ageing

The nurse's skills and knowledge of the ageing process are crucial in order to assess and intervene positively with the older person. Many of the most commonly seen health problems in older people are associated with age-related changes in the muscles, joints and bones. Although ageing alone does not need to restrict an individual's mobility, the impact of these changes affects an individual's speed, posture, strength, body image, independence and safety (Goldman, 1986). The older person's gait alters and, due to the reduction in hip rotation and knee flexion during the swing phase, the foot is a smaller distance from floor. This may be why many older people trip and fall. (Nelson, Hughes, Virjee et al., 1991). Impaired balance is often seen in older people. This can be attributed to a variety of causes, such as degenerative changes in the vestibular system in the brain, which may impair the ability to right oneself when balance is challenged. A reduction in the level of activity, rather than an actual age-related change, is thought to cause the changes in muscle strength (Rickli and Busch, 1986).

The ageing process affects the respiratory system and, in combination with often chronic lung disease, can cause shortness of breath, thus severely impairing a person's ability to walk unaided, or to exercise freely.

The risk of falling

An older person's posture tends to take on an attitude of general flexion, with the lumbar spine flattening, and the head tilting forward. Directly related to the changes in posture are those of body alignment, as ageing brings a shift in the body's gravity. Due to the tendency of the head to tilt forward and in front of the usual line of the centre of gravity, the older person is at increased risk of losing balance and thus falling.

Nurses must not overlook the effect of age-related changes in vision on an individual's ability to move freely with confidence. Any loss of vision can have a major impact on how older people manage their daily lives.

The risk of falls and injuries because of a failure to see obstacles or a changed environment, are much higher due to age-related changes in the iris and pupils. Less light is admitted to the retina, a process known as 'senile miosis' (Kolanowski, 1992). An older person therefore needs not only a greater amount of light in order to see effectively, but also more time to adjust to light changes. Moving from a dim room, or going outside at night, can temporarily cause visual difficulties and thus increase the risk of a fall.

Common disease processes in older people

There are a number of common disease processes in older people that have direct implications on movement ability. In order to effectively deliver the most appropriate care, the nurse has to understand the mechanisms of the disease process and its implications for the individual.

Pain

Whatever disease process is prevalent, pain is often the major problem in preventing an older person from being independent in movement. When it hurts to move, the most natural reaction is to stop activity. Many older people are reluctant to admit to feeling pain, or to request pain relief, possibly being frightened of the side-effects that can occur with analgesics, such as constipation or drowsiness. Everyone has a different pain threshold. Nurses should ensure that they respect the older person's perception of his or her own pain, and treat accordingly. It is also important to ensure that chronic pain is managed prophylactically and, if the person is to be encouraged to move, the nurse must make sure that all obstacles are removed.

Arthritis

Osteo arthritis and rheumatoid arthritis, especially of the lower limbs and spine, are a major cause of reduced mobility in older people, the main symptoms being pain and stiffness of the affected joints.

Osteoporosis

Osteoporosis which particularly affects older women, is a major cause of fractures, leading to hospital admission, loss of independence, and premature death. Osteoporosis of the rib cage and vertebrae can result in kyphosis, which not only accounts for an older person's stooped posture, but also makes walking, breathing deeply, and exercise more difficult.

Parkinson's disease

Parkinson's disease is a major movement disorder experienced by older people. The main symptoms are slowed movement (bradykinesia), rigidity, postural instability and tremors. A person with Parkinson's disease may experience hesitation in movement at particular times, e.g. passing through a doorway, or may freeze at certain times of the day. In a care home setting, the nurse plays a major role in monitoring on and off periods and ensuring that medication is administered at the appropriate times. For many people who experience Parkinson's disease, the period of the day when they are switched 'on', alert, and able to carry out independent activities, may not always be the socially acceptable time. For example they may wish to dust their room or do some personal washing in the middle of the night.

Cerebral vascular accidents

Many neurological events such as cerebral vascular accidents, or transient ischaemic attacks, have profound effects on an individual's ability to move and function independently, ranging from complete immobility through to an unsteady gait. The nurse must understand how these events can affect the individual, and the appropriate strategies to be used to maximise recovery and maintain independence.

Foot problems

Many older people have problems associated with foot disorders. There is a clear relationship between foot problems and the immobility of older people (Schank, 1987). The most prevalent problems which affect older people are corns, calluses, trouble with toenails, foot deformities resulting from badly-fitting shoes in youth, and arthritis. The nurse should accurately assess not only the state of the person's feet, but also their ability to care for their own feet. Many older people may be suffering from illnesses that make it difficult, or impossible, for them to cope with regular cleaning and care of their feet (Andrews, 1987).

Sudden reduction in an older person's mobility, or the 'off legs' syndrome

'Off legs' appears to have become a euphemistic phrase, commonly used by physicians, nurses, and many others who work with older people. It indicates that an individual who has previously been able to maintain a certain degree of independent movement has deteriorated to an extent that requires intervention/assistance. It is crucial to remember that this kind of episode is not a normal part of the ageing process. Older people do not automatically lose their mobility. This is invariably due to external factors, such as a disease process or other intervention. There are a number of predisposing factors that can cause a sudden loss of mobility in an older person. The nurse's role as the key professional in a care home setting is crucial. The nurse is able to take the appropriate preventative and proactive measures to prevent the older person from experiencing possible long-term detrimental effects of reduced mobility.

Infections are a major cause of this syndrome, particularly those of the chest and urinary tract. The symptoms of pyrexia, pain, and often confusion are early warning signs for which nurses should be on the lookout. Early detection and the appropriate treatment are crucial in ensuring that there are no long-term effects. An exacerbation of an existing condition, such as cardiac dysfunction, an extension of a stroke, or rheumatoid arthritis, can all precipitate an 'off legs' episode. The difficulty in adjusting to a sudden change in health status can be very distressing.

Drugs and mobility

Many older people suffer from complex, multi-pathology disease processes, necessitating a variety of drugs to be taken (polypharmacy), thus increasing the possibility of side-effects ad drug induced complications.

Drugs which affect postural stability, such as sedatives, hypnotics, and certain tranquillisers can have a very detrimental effect on an older person's ability to move independently. Of particular note is the drug nitrazepam (Mogadon), still commonly taken as night sedation by older people in this country. This has a half life of up to 60 hours, thus possibly causing drowsiness into the next day and consequent poor mobility (Swift, 1983).

Principles of rehabilitation in older people

Rehabilitation with older people is about being positive. It does not just take place in special units, but continues in the person's own home, in hospital, or in care homes. Older people have the potential to improve or maintain their health status, even if remaining highly dependent on others. All members of the team should participate in the process of enabling and facilitating older people to ensure they are able to achieve the maximum movement and mobility. The nurse's care plan should facilitate choice in a range of activities that encourages physical activity.

The nurse's role, working within the multi-disciplinary team in any care home setting, should aim to prevent any further loss of mobility, maintain and improve current ability, even on a very small scale, and should always be striving to enhance quality of life and preserve the dignity of the older person. In order to achieve these goals the nurse should have a working knowledge of the roles of the occupational therapist, physiotherapist, and chiropodist, in order to understand how their specialist skills can be used effectively to encourage good nursing practice. This will also ensure that accurate referral can be made for specialist services through the person's GP.

Health promotion in the community

In any care home setting, the nurse is the professional who is able to facilitate normal life activities. Education to enable the older person (and the carers) to manage any disability in the most positive manner is crucial.

Older people's requirements to remain as fit and active as possible are no different to those of younger people. An important element is access to regular exercise, coupled with sound nutrition. Offering an older person sufficient time to walk to the dining table for a meal, supported by a nurse if required, and without being rushed, can be as beneficial as arranging specific exercises classes. It can combine social interaction, motivation, nutrition and physical exercise to ensure muscle strength can be maintained. As inactivity can play a major part in causing the muscle weakness and lack of stamina commonly found in older people, regular exercise tailored to the individual is essential (Nokes, 1994). Recent research indicates that regular exercise can improve muscle strength even in the older person Fiatarone, Marks, Ryan, et al., 1990).

EXTEND is a registered charity, and is the name of a series of therapeutic exercises. Set to music, these have been designed particularly for older people, aiming to enhance their quality of life. EXTEND teachers can train nurses and other professionals allied to medicine. There are local classes all over the country and they are able to initiate groups within day centres and care homes. The community or hospital-based occupational therapy department or local hospital services for older people should be able to give more information.

Regular access to chiropody is crucial in maintaining mobility in older people. One of the aims of the chiropodist, whether in hospital or in the community, is to promote pain-free healthy feet and maintain the mobility of older people.

Promoting mobility through health promotion should include every aspect of the person's health status, and referral of advice from relevant specialists should be made whenever the nurse feels it is appropriate.

The dependency cycle and mobility

The nurse working in a care home setting will often be faced with caring for somebody who is highly dependent and who presents as highly dependent. Dependency does not always occur because someone has become physically unable to move or walk. The nurse should be aware of all parts of the programme of care and how each impacts on the older person in an institutional setting. One of the most important considerations is to ensure that the person has a purpose for his or her action or activity. Within normal life every action has a purpose whether to fulfil a task of daily living, or to bring pleasure, or fulfil a personal need. It is very easy within a care home setting for the nurse to carry out tasks for the older person in order to 'help them out', to 'save time' or because the nurse cannot sit back and encourage the older people to help themselves.

There is evidence to suggest that nurses can cause dependency simply by the method of care adopted in the care environment. It has been shown that task allocation forces more dependency than primary nursing, as every action is a task and not a part of the total care package (Miller, 1985). This can be illustrated by looking at the negative effect a nurse can have on an older person by reinforcing dependency.

An elderly lady with arthritis in her knee, who is mildly confused and has a continence problem, is admitted to a care home as her husband can no longer cope. Although disabled, she could do a small amount of housework and would always get up and fetch the paper from the front door. In the home, the nurses would bring the paper to her bed, instead of helping and encouraging her to walk to collect it. As a result she sits for longer, starts to lose interest and dozes more. Her self-esteem is lowered, she does not take exercise, and so her joints stiffen. This increases the pain and her reluctance to move. As she dozes more, her sleep pattern is disturbed and she becomes more confused. Her mood becomes lower as she feels she has no value, and so her appetite deteriorates. With lowered nutritional intake, low mood, poor sleep and immobility, there is a greater risk of a pressure sore and more work for the care staff.

Not only has the lady become dependent on the nurses, but the nurses have increased the work load within that home simply because the lady was not assessed and treated holistically. Explanation and encouragement should be offered and the person should be supported and encouraged to continue the level of activity they can achieve.

Psychological and interpersonal skills used in managing a person's mobility

In order to ensure older people reach their optimum level of independence, or that they do not deteriorate, it is important to establish not only what physical care and rehabilitation can be undertaken, but the psychological and interpersonal care that can also be given. The impact of the downward spiral has been demonstrated. An integral part of this is the lowered self-esteem of the person and feeling of poor self-worth. Some physical illnesses such as Parkinson's disease, strokes and endocrine disorders, are known to cause clinical depression (Burn and Dearden, 1990). The symptoms, including low mood, loss of interest, change of diurnal variation in a person's mood and reduced energy, should always be dealt with and assessed by an appropriately qualified person. These symptoms can also present themselves in a person who is not feeling valued, or who is feeling worthless, thus reinforcing the dependency cycle. There are a number of interpersonal skills the nurse can adopt to help prevent the dependency cycle impacting on the older person. Use yourself as a therapeutic tool.

Being positive

An older person is more aware than anybody of the impact of his or her disability. Look for ways of doing things differently or more easily for the person, in order for them to succeed and be in control. Be positive, but not patronising in the language used to praise and encourage the person. This can be achieved by talking with the person about how best to move or change position.

Using nonverbal communication

Messages are transmitted by the spoken word, the tone of the voice used, and the body movement and postures adopted. It is important that the nurse is aware of all the messages that are being communicated between the patient and the nurse and what those messages say. Be aware of the older person's personal space. For example for some people, being held around the shoulders is overpowering and disconcerting (Langland and Panicucci, 1982). Even how close the nurse stands to older people to encourage them to move or walk, if not clearly explained, may cause distress, because the accepted level of personal space (that is the boundary between two people) will vary with the relationship of the two people and also with the culture of that person (Pease, 1984). The intimate zone for Europeans is about 15–46 cm around the body, but for other cultures it is wider. Although close contact may be necessary to help somebody move, the reasons should be explained through verbal and non-verbal communication. Messages need to be clear. For example, if the nurse wants the older person to put on his or her own clothes and make positive statements but then, when the older person takes a little while over the task, stands over the person whilst leaning against the wall in a dominant fashion, this will intimidate the resident and reduce their self-confidence (Pease, 1984).

Use touch in a productive way

In childhood touch is a means of learning and discovering. As a person ages, the use of touch changes, and in older people expressive touch is dramatically reduced. Nurses touch predominantly in order to carry out physical tasks (MacLeod-Clarke, 1983). Touch communicates caring and empathy. For the person to be able to touch increases their spatial awareness. The sensory stimulation received through touch acts to comfort, to reassure, and to transmit information. Any surface that interferes with the direct interface between the person's skin and the object will reduce the amount of information received. For example a person in a wheelchair does not perceive the feeling of movement in the same way as the ambulatory patient (Hollinger, 1980). Residents should be encouraged therefore to feel and touch and, if they appear to grab or grasp at staff, a reassuring approach should be taken in order to support them. Nurses should take opportunities to hold the patient's hand and stimulate tactile senses with gentle massage.

Value the person, their beliefs and their wishes, at the centre of any care plan

It is easy for nurses to look at the needs of the resident and make judgements about what parts of the person's mobility and movement should be prioritised for maintaining. However, the nurse should balance the clinical needs against what the resident may desire in order to feel more personally fulfilled. The beliefs, wishes and cultural or religious value systems should be held in equal importance for the older person. A

Muslim man who has Parkinson's disease may find kneeling difficult; patterns of care should be developed in order to help him kneel and bow to the floor when at prayer. For a Hindu person it may be important to be able to stand up long enough to wash in running water, yet for a retired business executive who has always played golf, he may wish to be able to continue going out from the care setting in order to have a drink at the bar of his club. The value system of the older person should be central to the mobility plan devised. This should also be reflected in the actions undertaken by nurses and the respect shown for cultural beliefs. In particular, nurses should acknowledge these in touch, physical contact, clothing and by viewing the older person within the family unit.

Balancing therapy, humanity and safety in the care environment

Care home settings are environments where three life styles converge. The nurse enters this place of work and has to conduct their professional practice as effectively as possible. The host organisation has to ensure the care is of a high quality, that safety is maintained: that the building is clean and presentable, and that the budgetary requirements are met. For the older person the care home is the setting whether their past, present and future may confront them. The role of the nurse is to marry these three very different needs in a painless, seamless way, ensuring that all three interested parties (or stake holders) maintain equal importance. The fabric of the setting must be pleasing firstly to the older person who has to live there. It must resemble their home; every generation and every culture develops styles appropriate to them. Individual influence on the decor can help the person feel more involved. A number of areas of the fabric of the building directly affect a person's mobility and a nurse should consider the impact these areas have on all three stake holders when involved in any planning or purchasing arrangement.

Floor covering

In the UK the modern desirable floor covering is carpet. In care home environments it is still not automatically the choice, particularly in corridors and bedrooms, because of problems of hygiene and friction on the older person's shoes or walking aids causing difficulty in walking. However, evidence suggests that older people walk faster and more confidently on carpet then on vinyl floor (Wilmott, 1986). There is also some thought that there are less falls on carpet and injuries are less severe than falls on vinyl covered floors (Healey, 1994). Cleaning and hygiene routines can eliminate difficulties with odour. Rugs and loose mats, however, should be discouraged as they can easily be tripped over. Similarly, nurses must be aware of difficulties older people may have as floor surfaces change. People with an intention tremor or those with perceptual disturbance may have difficulty in judging the change in texture, and thus overbalance or fall.

Lighting

Lighting in all rooms should be chosen carefully. Fluorescent central lights are bright and clear but may cause problems for older people with visual difficulties as they can be too bright. Subdued wall lighting may equally cast shadows, or reduce peoples visibility. Both extremes will affect the confidence of somebody with mobility problems (Kolanowski, 1992).

Wall covering

It is important to always anticipate the impact of all types of stimulation on mobility. Older people who lack confidence or energy may find that corridors decorated in horizontal patterns or large printed paper are quite exhausting. Colours should be chosen that are warm and encouraging, and toilet and bathroom doors should be painted in a primary colour in order to help the older person plan his or her journey and see where they are heading.

Furniture

Traditional furniture for older people is plastic-covered high-backed chairs, often that tilt backwards. This outdated image is no longer appropriate or necessary. With good continence management, all residents should have a cloth or 'normal' fabric chair and tipping people back only causes more confusion and agitation. For many patients this is disorientating and counter-productive. Lounge chairs should be supportive with arms, and the room should have a variety of heights so that each older person can find a chair that is an equal height to their lower leg. This assists with ejection when the person wants to get up. Settees, although often lower, aid communication and create a more domestic environment, thereby improving the milieu and raising the self-esteem of the residents (Phair and Good, 1989). Dining-room furniture should always be provided with carver chairs in order to offer the person support as he or she stands and also help in stabilising somebody when sitting if their balance is impaired.

Beds and mattreses

In order to create a homely environment, divan beds are frequently used in care home settings. These may, however, be too low for a person to get up. Equally, a hospital bed may be too high for the person to touch the ground. The nurse should ensure that each person is assessed, and that an appropriate height bed is found. This problem is made worse is pressure sore relieving overlay mattresses are added to the height of the bed. This should be considered when equipment is purchased. For some older people a replacement mattress system would be safer and assist with mobility.

Assisting with independence

Handrails along all corridors and regular seating should be available. Small journeys will encourage older people to be mobile, as they will be rewarded for these achievements. If the seating is placed by a window or is made to be attractive it will again give a positive message of success. Toilets should be large enough to take a walking frame, or a wheelchair and a nurse. Seats should, where possible be raised.

A person who has mobility problems should be given small goals to achieve. Many care home settings are large buildings. Encouragement should be given to the person to walk, but within reason. If a person wishes to go to the toilet, it may be better for that person if they are taken there quickly in a wheelchair, and then encouraged to walk back at their leisure. It is tempting in a busy unit to always use a chair rather than walk with the person but, as already demonstrated, that it not necessarily the most appropriate course of action in the long term.

Lifting and manual handling

Lifting people has always been considered by nurses an integral part of their role as a carer; and subsequent back injuries have often been considered one of the hazards of the job. However, in January 1993, new health and safety regulations on the minimum requirements of loads were introduced. The legislation was effected in order to implement the European directives (HSE, 1991). Lifting appropriately is now, therefore, a statutory requirement, and nurses, alongside managers, have a professional obligation to ensure that appropriate skills are learned or revised. Changing practice is not always easy, and some staff who practice traditional methods of care may find it difficult to immediately take on new ideas. Peer group pressure to conform to old ways has been found as a reason why staff with new skills sometimes give in to tradition. It has been found that, in order to introduce new lifting practice into the workplace, it is important that the nurse had knowledge, skills, assertiveness, confidence, and a belief in good nursing practice (Kane and Parahoo, 1994). For these reasons it is important to support nurses who are trying to improve lifting techniques in all settings.

Risk factors

All nurses should ensure that an appropriate lifting assessment is undertaken and all risk factors are considered:

● the patient's weight, an obvious factor, should be measured accurately and 8 stone or 50 kg is judged to be the maximum that two staff should lift without a hoist;
● the person's mobility, and how much they can assist the nurse;
● their height compared to those of the nurses;
● if the person is mentally alert and willing to help, or if they are confused;

- if the person has any motor neurone problems;
- if the nurse and carers helping are trained in lifting techniques; and
- if the room is well designed.

There are now lifting assessments designed for a quick but effective assessment of the patient's needs. These should be incorporated into all care plans (Pilling, 1993), and all staff encouraged to follow the identified plan.

Using appropriate equipment and lifting techniques

Lifting equipment has been available for many years. For many nurses, however, there has been either an inherent dislike of this, or a belief that it was unnecessary or uncomfortable for the patient. Nurses can no longer afford to carry such prejudices. Lifting equipment is as vital in a care setting as any other piece of health care equipment. With the implementation of the manual handling regulations, some lifting techniques were made illegal and condemned. These included the technique where one nurse was either side of the person moving them up the bed as the nurse is too far away from the patient and the weight is borne by the back. Also the underarm drag lift is condemned as the nurse's body twists. This also puts sheer forces on the patient's skin and pulls up their arms or shoulders. The Australian lift is still considered the safest and most appropriate lift to use for people in bed.

There are more than 60 different hoists and 150 slings available (Stacey, 1994). Because of the wide variety of lifting equipment available, it is advisable for a nurse to discuss his or her requirements with a lifting expert before purchasing equipment, so that the most appropriate choice for their unit can be made. Some hoists lift someone into the upright position, some hold them in a sitting one. Lifting belts are very useful for helping people to stand or be moved up the bed. A turning sheet assists with the movement of a very immobile person in bed, and a turning board helps a nurse working alone to move a person from one chair to another. Hoists can be manual or electric, static or mobile, and come in a variety of sizes. Some are so versatile that they can be carried in the boot of a car. Expert advice should be sought, however, to ensure that the correct equipment is purchased for the correct environment.

Ergonomics

It is important that all lifting is conducted as safely as possible. Safety can be ensured by applying the principles of ergonomics, that is assessing the work place, the environment, how the work is organised and the social environment (McAtamney and Hignett, 1993). In practice this means that the nurse should assess everything around him or her to ascertain how best to approach the problem. Examples might include:

- moving any furniture that prevents the nurse bending, e.g. a locker;
- loosening their own tight clothing;
- checking that the floor is not wet and that the working space is clear;

- checking if the lighting is adequate to enable the nurse to see what is happening;
- checking if the nurse can get an appropriate grip;
- checking if the bed is at its lowest point; and
- ascertaining if the patient is able to understand what is going to happen to him or her, and applying good communication skills.

This small list of examples can be added to ad infinitum. As well as deciding if all ergonomic factors have been applied, it is also important to assess whether the ergonomic principle of reducing the need to lift or move the person could be applied.

- Use dynamic flotation systems for very ill people who are at high risk from pressure sores, to reduce the amount of manual handling required.
- Give a person a monkey pole or a P bar to enable them to move themselves.
- Use loose fitting clothing (within the style approved by the patient) to make moving easier.
- Reassess the person's medication to ensure none are causing unnecessary muscle spasm or stiffness.

Lifting and manual handling regulations/principles also quite obviously apply to inert objects, and to repetitive activities that might put a strain on the back. Trolleys or wheelchairs should be used whenever possible to move any object that feels heavy to the nurse. A step stool should be used to reach very high cupboards, and perhaps the introduction of duvets instead of heavy blankets would help to reduce repetitive strain. Under the new regulations, employers have a duty to provide adequate equipment and apply ergonomic principles in the workplace. Employees also have a duty to use appropriate techniques and ergonomic principles in order to reduce the danger of damage to both the nurse and the patient.

Conclusion

For many older people living in a care home setting, the goal of maintaining or restoring independent movement is central to their quality of life. The often complex, multiple causes of reduced mobility in an older person require a holistic approach within the multi-disciplinary framework. The nurse's role within this team is to work towards preventing any further loss of mobility, while maintaining and, if possible, improving their current ability, if this is what the older person wishes. The nurse who can combine a knowledge of the ageing process, an understanding of how disease can affect the older person, the effect of the environment, and issues around health promotion, with accurate assessment skills, is thus uniquely placed to perform this role. If the nurse if aware of his or her own communication skills, and the needs and desires of the older person, coupled with any psychological distress they may be experiencing, positive interventions can be achieved. Working in partnership with the older person, the nurse can assist in whatever way is valued by the patient, to immeasurably enhance the quality of life.

References

Andrews, K. (1987) *Foot Disorders, Rehabilitation of the Older Adult.* Edward Arnold.

Burn, W. and Dearden, T. (1990) Physical Aspects of Depression. *Geriatric Medicine,* May, 61–64.

Farquhar, M., Grundy, E and Formby, J. (1993) Functional Ability of Very Elderly People. *Nursing Standard,* **7,** 51, 31–36.

Fiatarone, M.A., and Marks, E.C., Ryan, N.D., Meredith, C.N., Lipsitz, L.A. and Evans, W.J. (1990) High intensity strength training in nonagenarians. Effects on skeletal muscle. *Journal of the American Medical Association,* **26,** 3029–3034.

Goldman, R. (1986) Ageing Changes in Structure and Function. In D. Carnevali and M. Patrick (ed.) *Nursing Management for the Eldery.* J B Lippincott.

Healey, F. (1994) Does flooring type affect risk of injury in older patients? *Nursing Times,* **90,** 27, 40–41.

Health and Safety Executive (1991) *The Manual Handling of Loads. Proposals for Regulations and Guidance.* HMSO.

Hollinger L. (1980) Perception of Touch in the Elderly. *Journal of Gerontological Nursing,* **6,** 12, 741–746.

Kane, R.A. and Kane, R.L. (1988) *Assessing the Elderly. A Practical Guide to Measurement.* Lexicon, MA: Lexicon Books.

Kane, M. and Parahoo, K. (1994) Lifting. Why Nurses follow Bad Practice. *Nursing Standard,* **8,** 25, 34–38.

Kolanowski, A.M. (1992) The clinical importance of environmental lighting in the elderly. *Journal of Gerontological Nursing,* **18,** 1, 10.

Langland, R. and Panicucci, C. (1982) Effects of Touch on communication with elderly confused clients. *Journal of Gerontological Nursing,* **8,** 3, 152–155.

MacLeod-Clarke, J. (1983) Nurse Patient Communication. An analysis of conversations from Surgical Wards. *Nursing Research: Ten Studies in Patient Care.* John Wiley.

McAtamney, L. and Hignett, S. (1993) A space to move in. *Nursing Times,* **89,** 18, 44–46.

Miller, A. (1985) Nurse/Patient dependency. Is it iatrogenic? *Journal of Advanced Nursing,* **10,** 63–69.

Nelson, P., Huges, S. and Virjee, S. et al. (1991) Walking speed as a measure of disability. *Care of the Elderly,* **3,** 3, 125–126.

Nokes, K.M. (1994) Activity Exercise Pattern in Care-planning for the Older Adult. In R. Ferri (ed.) *Nursing diagnosis in Long Term Care.* W B Saunders.

Pease, A. (1984) *Body Langauge.* Oxford University Press.

Phair, L. and Good, E. (1989) People not patients. *Nursing Times*, **85**, 23, 42–44.

Pilling, S. (1993) Calculating the Risk. *Nursing Standard*, **8**, 634–638.

Rickli, R. and Busch, S. (1986) Motor performance of women as a function of age and physical activity level. *Journal of Gerontology*, **41**, 645–649.

Schrank, N.J. (1987) A Survey of the Well Elderly. Their foot problems, practices and needs. *Journal of Gerontological Nursing*, **3**, 11, 151.

Stacey, N. (1994) Moving People. *Nursing Times*, **90**, 19, 47–50.

Swift, C.G. (1983) Hypnotic drugs. In B. Isaacs (ed.) *Recent Advances in Geriatric Medicine*. Churchill Livingstone.

Wilmott, M. (1986) The effect of vinyl floor surface and a carpeted floor surface upon walking in elderly hospital inpatients. *Age and ageing*, **15**, 119–120.

14

Continence

Hilary Oliver and Pauline Ford

Introduction

Nurses take the lead in continence promotion and can greatly influence the quality of life for older people. A recent study showed that 57 per cent of residents in nursing homes in England are continent (DoH, 1992), yet despite this continence or the symptoms of incontinence feature significantly in the work of nurses who provide services for older people. This is particularly the case when the older person requires care of a continuing nature, such as that given in care homes and other settings which provide continuous nursing.

It is therefore highly appropriate that nurses develop both the knowledge and skills required for the promotion of continence and the resolution of symptoms of incontinence where this is achievable. Such expertise will not only impact on quality of life but is also likely to be cost effective, particularly when it reduces the need for incontinence aids and equipment.

This chapter considers how the ageing process affects continence and why some older people become incontinent. It describes the nurse's role in undertaking comprehensive assessment of an older person and planning care and treatment. Finally it suggests strategies for continence promotion and management.

Age-related changes associated with continence

The causes of incontinence are complex and must be viewed alongside other aspects of physical and mental well-being. Ageing can present some challenges and one of these may be incontinence.

Age-related changes affect the ability of the kidneys to concentrate urine and maintain PH (acid/alkali) balance. Other age-related changes result in greater volumes of urine being produced, particularly at night. There is a greater risk of dehydration as the kidneys are less able to concentrate urine and preserve fluid. It has been suggested (Rowe, 1988) that age-related arteriosclerotic changes give rise to reduced blood flow, resulting in less efficient working of the kidneys.

As with renal function, so ageing affects bladder function in both men and women. The bladder epthelium becomes thinner. The bladder becomes less compliant and the capacity may be reduced; the bladder is not able to hold as much urine and does not relax as well during filling.

Ageing affects the amount of both sensory and motor impulses which influence bladder emptying. The older person may not be aware that the bladder is filling up until it is 90 per cent full. This may well result in them having less time than a younger person to reach the toilet in time to pass urine.

Incontinence can therefore result. The closing pressure of the urethra diminishes in older women which, it is suggested, might be related to the replacement of the smooth muscle by collagen. Oestrogen depletion may also affect the urethral closure mechanism leading to stress incontinence. Lack of oestrogen may cause urethritis, symptoms of which are similar to cystitis: frequency and urgency. On examination this condition may be easily seen as an inflamed red, often dry vulval area and is known as atrophic or senile vaginitis.

Men's prostate glands enlarge with age. The incidence of malignancy increases with age and may present in as many as 80 per cent of men aged over 90 years. Most of these malignancies are latent and do not affect life expectancy, but undoubtedly, the efficient emptying of the bladder is affected. Prostatic enlargement, both benign and malignant, can lead to an increased amount of residual urine because of urethral obstruction. Residual urine can cause a blackflow to the kidneys resulting in damage and infection. Older men are at risk of urinary tract infection.

The majority of older people remain continent all their lives but are more susceptible to incontinence than younger people because of the additional pathological, physiological, pharmacological and psychological factors from which they are at risk. Older people are likely to cope with such challenges as long as they remain in familiar surroundings and circumstances.

Potential causes of incontinence

Environmental

When an older person moves into a care home he or she will need time to adjust. Different routines, remembering where the toilet is, asking for help, sharing the same facilities, possibly with people of the opposite sex, will inevitably be different. The height of a chair, and being able to climb in and out of bed, are important issues to consider. There should be sufficient toilets which are well lit and easily found and accessed. They should be designed to accommodate the individual, associated walking aids, wheelchairs and staff as required. Extra rails, raised toilet seats, good lighting and reachable toilet paper will all enhance the ability to retain independence and thus promote continence.

Those from different cultural backgrounds may need special toilet facilities, which clearly should be identified before the individual moves into the home. For example, Muslims may wish to wash the vulval, perineal and anal areas each time the toilet is used and therefore need washing facilities in the toilet cubicle with some means of pouring water directly onto themselves. If a commode or urinal is used then washing facilities must be offered. Hindus may also wish to wash after using the toilet.

Physical changes

Coping with bladder and bowel function may be difficult for those who are experiencing other challenges associated with ageing. For example, regular eye tests should be undertaken to ensure optimal vision; treatable eye problems such as cataracts and glaucoma can be detected early and treated. Older people who can walk to the toilet independently are less likely to experience incontinence than those who require assistance. Reduced hearing which affects communication, and, poor dexterity which affects management of personal clothing and inappropriate footwear will all potentially impact on the older person's ability to physically control their toileting requirements. Mobility rather than cognitive impairment has been demonstrated to be the crucial predictor for continence amongst nursing home residents (Jirovec and Wells, 1990).

Types of incontinence

Stress incontinence

Stress incontinence results in a small amount of leakage on physical exertion such as coughing, laughing or sneezing. It normally affects women but can affect men after some surgery, i.e. trans urethral resection of the prostate (TURP). It is caused by incompetent urethra closure mechanisms and is common in pregnant and post menopausal women as the urethra becomes less elastic.

Urgency and urge incontinence

This is caused by a lack of ability to suppress a bladder contraction. The resident will complain of having to rush to the toilet urgently and will often leak urine if they do not get to the toilet in time (urge incontinence).

Urge incontinence results in the leakage of urine often in quite large amounts. Frequency will often be experienced. Sometimes the location of toilets are such a distance away that the individual may seem unusually keen to sit almost outside the toilet permanently in an effort to get to it in time.

Voiding disorders

Paradoxically some people develop continence problems because they cannot empty their bladder completely. By far the most common reason for this is outflow obstruction in men caused by an enlarged prostate gland. Men may first notice a slowing in the rate at which they pass urine, and the need to go more often to the toilet. They may develop symptoms of urgency, frequency and nocturia. These symptoms are all caused by the incomplete emptying of the bladder, so that a residual volume builds up, bringing an increased risk of urinary tract infections.

Voiding disorders may also be caused by inadequate detrusor contractions, sometimes known as detrusor failure, or atonic bladder. The sufferers are usually women. They may be completely unaware of the gradual build up of a residual volume of urine, only realising there is a problem when leakage starts to occur. It is a chronic condition with many underlying causes such as diabetic neuropathy or other neurological disease.

The presenting symptoms may be similar to those of urgency and frequency in that the sufferer will complain of having to go to the toilet frequently. However on close questioning, the client will describe frequent visits to the toilet, often timed by the clock, as a somewhat desperate attempt to avoid episodes of incontinence. The significant difference here is that the individual does not describe an urgent response to the recognised need to void urine. Dribbling incontinence may also occur, sometimes only at night. The most effective accurate assessment is to measure the residual volume of urine (see Assessment section, below).

Constipation also causes difficulty with the voiding of urine. A loaded rectum will partially occlude the bladder outlet, causing inefficient emptying.

Older people may develop what is known as a 'neurogenic bladder'. The term describes a reduced bladder capacity, increased residual volumes of urine, and uncontrolled bladder contractions (Norton, 1986). In other other words, the bladder will not store very much urine and will empty inefficiently with little warning. Neurological diseases associated with old age such as Parkinson's disease, and cerebrovascular accidents will affect efficient bladder sensation and voiding.

Nocturia

Arousal from sleep to pass urine, and night time incontinence are common problems among older people. This has been referred to in an earlier section but clearly nurses need to to respond to this in terms of clinical practice at night.

Medication

Drugs may well precipitate incontinence. The most obvious problems can be caused by diuretics. Loop diuretics such as frusemide are powerful and cause the bladder to fill rapidly, giving the person little time to respond. Night sedation will dull the senses, giving rise to night time incontinence. Some antidepressants, such as amitriptyline and imipramine may cause difficulty with micturition because of their effect on the smooth muscle of the bladder wall. Analgesics, particularly codeine and opiates, cause constipation.

In fact, many drugs affect bladder function and it is always worth checking the side-effects. Older people do not metabolise drugs as quickly as younger people and there may be a gradual build up of side effects. Also, combinations of drugs such as night sedation followed by an early morning dose of a diuretic will almost inevitably result in incontinence. A review of medications therefore should always be conducted. It is also important to recognise incontinence which suddenly presents and which may therefore be associated with new prescriptions (see Chapter 16).

Faecal incontinence

Whilst it is less common than urinary incontinence, nurses who work with older people will know that its incidence causes challenges for both the individual and the nurse. There are three principal causes: faecal impaction, neurological disease and diarrhoea (McClymont, Thomas and Denham, 1991).

Faecal impaction is not uncommon, and is the direct result of constipation. Where there is a slowing down of the passage of faeces, excess fluid is removed, and the faeces harden. This can impact in the rectum and, in response excessive amounts of mucus are produced. The individual becomes unaware of the loaded rectum and does not experience a desire to defaecate. Above the impaction, faeces become liquefied by bacterial action. These faeces pass around the impacted stool and present as spurious diarrhoea. It is not uncommon for anti-diarrhoeal prescriptions to be administered, which of course results in a worsening of the situation. Eventually the client is likely to become anorexic, will vomit and exhibit very restless behaviour.

Assessment

For the individual, incontinence is embarrassing, causing loss of self esteem and dignity. One study demonstrated that even when individuals admit to the problem, they do not necessarily want to seek the assistance of a nurse or doctor (O'Brien, Austin, Sethi and O'Boyle, 1991). Significant skill and perception is therefore required on the part of the nurse. Sensitivity and tact is essential if an effective outcome is to be achieved (Moody 1990). The key to successful outcomes lies in assessment undertaken by a nurse or doctor who has knowledge, skill, time and sensitivity resulting in genuine compassion for the individual. Assessment begins with:

- interview and discussion,
- physical examination,
- investigations,
- continence charts, and
- multi-disciplinary approaches.

The use of an assessment tool or check list standardises the care team's approach (Duffin, 1992). It also enables all members of the care team to use the information in a unified way and ensures that there is consistency of approach.

Interview

Nurses are often the ones to identify urinary incontinence but nurses and doctors have historically been very passive in its treatment (Ebersole and Hess, 1990). Assessment is multi-dimensional. It should include a health history, physical examination, laboratory analysis and in exceptional circumstances urodynamic evaluations. It should also include predisposing factors such as environmental influences.

The nurse should obtain a thorough health history which can assist the General Practitioner in making an accurate diagnosis. First of all, try to encourage the resident to describe their problem in their own words. Time will be of key importance so make sure that you are not going to be frequently interrupted. Sensitive assessments such as these may be best carried out once a resident has acclimatised to the care home and got to know the nurses a little. Obviously this may not always be possible but do bear in mind that incontinence is a 'taboo' subject for some people. Positive and sensitive responses are obviously required. Saying 'never mind' or 'it doesn't matter' gives the wrong signals when, almost certainly, it matters profoundly to the older person, even if they appear quite dismissive or nonchalant about it. Talk about helping the individual to regain continence.

Assessment data should include the duration, frequency, and volume of the incontinence. Specific questions should be asked about voiding patterns and when and where episodes of leakage occur. Accurate detail should be collected relating to any symptoms of burning, itching or pressure. The character of the urine (odour, colour, cloudy or clear) and any difficulty in starting or stopping the urinary stream all need to be recorded.

Information about the past medical history should be noted along with any surgical procedures conditions which may influence neurological health. Women should be asked about their obstetric and gynaecological history.

Activities of daily living, ability to reach and/or find a toilet, and finger and wrist dexterity (affecting the management of clothing) should be documented.

Use of medications such as sedatives, hypnotics, anticholinergics, and antidepressants should be assessed. Frusemide, diazepam, amitryptiline and phenothiazines are among common drugs prescribed.

Don't forget to ask about the presence of discharges in both men and women and check the normal bowel movement patterns. In particular ask if there has been any constipation or diarrhoea.

Observation by all members of the team is also an important method of collecting information, and everyone should be encouraged to report to the registered nurse.

Physical examination

A registered nurse is likely to carry out some of the physical examination but must recognise when there is a need to obtain the expertise of the continence advisor and/or the GP. Any examination should include an assessment of mental state; mobility; dexterity; and a neurologic, abdominal, rectal and pelvic examination.

Physical examination may reveal a loaded rectum which once treated can often resolve incontinence of a transient nature. The observation of the vulval and perineal area in women may reveal senile vaginitis. The area will look red and will cause irritation. The women should be asked to cough and the presence of prolapse or leakage noted.

The contribution of the doctor will be needed to identify a cystocele in women and an enlarged prostate in men.

Investigations

Laboratory measurements should include urine analysis, serum creatinine or blood urea nitrogen and, as necessary, urine culture, blood sugar and urine cytology. The measurement of the residual volume of urine should be discussed with the doctor. It may be achieved by catheterisation or, preferably, by the use of ultrasound. Some continence advisors have access to a portable ultrasound. Routine tests should be carried out and a midstream specimen of urine sent to the laboratory. Whippo and Creason (1989) found that many older women had bacteruria which did not give rise to the accepted recognisable symptom of pyrexia and dysuria, etc., and the incidence rose among cognitively impaired women. Only 18 per cent of incontinent residents in their study were free of urinary tract infection.

Baseline continence charts

Information obtained by charting episodes of normal continence and episodes of incontinence complements information collected by interview and examination. The best person to fill in the chart is the resident. If this is not possible, then all members of the team should be encouraged to record accurately for about a week. It may be useful to measure each episode of voiding but that may be difficult. Simple ticks in each column for urine output and episodes of incontinence plus some sign for bowel movement and fluid intake and will provide valuable information. Many companies who market products for continence care will provide charts free of charge.

Contribution of other members of the team

Noting data during the assessment process will enable the nurse to report relevant details to other members of the team. The doctor is required for physical examinations and/or to consider changes in medication. A physiotherapist will be able to offer advice regarding specific exercises to assist in the management or resolution of incontinence, and an occupational therapist should be able to offer advice regarding management of clothing if dexterity is a problem.

Some nurses may find it helpful to use a checklist for the assessment of incontinence though this should be used discretely. In particular it may offer some useful information for the continence advisor or indeed the nurse who has gone on to undertake further education and training in continence promotion. An example of such a checklist is shown in Figure 14.1.

Resident reported, relative/staff reported

Onset
Past medical history
Past surgical history
Urinary symptoms
    Urgency
    Urge incontinence
    Frequency
    Stress incontinence
    No sensation of leakage
Bowel function
    Frequency, e.g. daily
    Consistency
    Difficulty in passing

Physical examination
Palpable bladder
Palpable faeces

Female
    Senile vaginitis
    Uterine prolapse
    Stress leakage

Male
    Hernia
    Prostatic enlargement

Rectal examination
    Presence of faeces
    Consistency of stool
    Haemorrhoids

Urine tests and dates
    Routine
    MSU
    Residual volume of urine

Baseline continence chart

Figure 14.1   *Assessment checklist for continence*

Based on the four components of assessment, a decision can be made regarding treatment or the need for further investigation. Accurate assessment can identify incontinence which is:

- **transient**, the result of temporary conditions that are amenable to medication, surgery, psychological support, and alternations to environmental factors, medications or clothing, or
- **established**, the result of neurological damage to the nervous system.

Transient incontinence is curable. Established incontinence is treatable or controllable.

Planning care and treatment

Planning care for continence promotion is a skilled activity. It requires application of knowledge, skills and sensitive observation of factors which may be contributing to continence. Making appropriate changes in care to resolve those problems may take time and will involve all members of the team.

Urgency and urge incontinence

May be resolved by reviewing the continence chart and making appropriate changes to times of visits to the toilet. The team must all understand that a request to go to the toilet should be responded to as quickly as possible in order to avoid urge incontinence. Location and access to toilets may need adjustment and the resident may need to be moved nearer a toilet to reduce anxiety. Always try to involve the resident in devising their toilet plan if at all possible.

Researchers have found that, 'two hourly toileting' does not achieve continence as an overall plan for a Nursing Home. Jilek (1993) describes trying to reduce incontinence in this way and admits lack of success. Burgio, McCormick, Sheve et al. (1994) also describes the lack of success with two hourly toileting. However,they describe great success with individual appropriately-timed, prompted visits to the toilet and success with telling each person when they will next be taken to the toilet. He found that residents no longer felt the need to make frequent, often inappropriate requests for staff assistance.

The timing of drug administration may be changed in order to avoid episodes of urgency at difficult times. For example, some residents may enjoy having breakfast in bed, so taking diuretics would be more appropriate for them later in the morning.

Stress incontinence

Contrary to popular belief, older women can improve symptoms of stress incontinence by doing pelvic floor exercises. Nurses can teach these exercises very effectively, following a pelvic floor assessment. A continence advisor can determine the strength, or otherwise, of a pelvic floor contraction by a digital vaginal examination (Brink, Sampselle, Wells, et al., 1989; Laycock, 1992). This will also help women identify the muscles to exercise. The index and middle finger should be inserted, and the woman asked to squeeze and lift, holding for ten seconds. After a minute, she should be asked to repeat the squeeze, and again as often as possible. The muscle strength is assessed using the Oxford grading system:

0: for no contraction
up to 5: strong contraction
The hold time is noted in seconds.

For example, a woman with a weak contraction held for three seconds would score 2 ÷ 3. The number of times she could repeat the contraction gives the final score – say four times. Final score 2 ÷ 3 × 4. All this information is then used to design an individual exercise plan, repeated eight times a day. Again, using the above example, the woman would perform two three-second contractions four times a session, with a minute's rest between each contraction (Laycock, 1992). So she would do 2 × 4 × 8 = 64 contractions every day of 3 seconds' duration.

Pelvic floor exercises should only follow skilled and expert assessment.

Teaching pelvic floor exercises

Having identified the muscles to exercise during assessment, the exercises may be described as follows:

1. Contract the posterior pelvic floor muscles as if trying to prevent passing wind from the anus.
2. Contract the anterior pelvic floor muscles as if trying to stop the flow of urine.

Voiding Disorders

Management of these difficulties will almost certainly require the expertise of a specialist. The opinion of a urologist may be required for a man with an outlet obstruction in treating him with surgery or, if surgery cannot be performed, then catheterisation may be the only option. There is a choice of urethral indwelling or intermittent catheterisation or supra pubic catheterisation. Chronic retention may be managed with occasional intermittent catheterisation. The help and advice of a Continence Advisor may be required to work out a suitable regime for an individual resident. Sometimes, the problem gradually resolves, for example as the resident's general health improves following orthopaedic surgery. In order to detect improvement, measurement of the amount of urine withdrawn on catheterisation should be continued.

Implementation

The implementation of care involves the whole team of carers, from the domestic staff who may be giving drinks and meals to residents to care assistants who may be taking the resident to the toilet, to report on progress.

It is important to maintain records and charts, particularly in the early stages of implementaion. In this way, evaluation becomes constructive, and further possible action can take place as a result. For example, if mesures to reduce episodes of urgency and urge incontinence are not very successful, then a small dose of an anticholinergic drug such as oxybutynin may be prescribed by the doctor.

Anticholinergic drugs reduce smooth muscle activity, in this case that of the detrusor. Unfortunately, they also affect other smooth muscles with the consequent side-effects of a dry mouth and constipation. Oxybutynin in doses of 2.5–5 mg can be taken to target times of day or a particular occasion, when problems of frequency and urgency would otherwise prevent the sufferer taking part in something they wish to do.

Constipation

The accepted definition of constipation is 'the difficult and infrequent passage of a hard stool'. This can be a misleading definition as there may well be colonic faecal loading of quite soft stool, particularly in older people who have mobility difficulties. The common causes of constipation are:

- immobility;
- dehydration;
- inadequate diet;
- ano-rectal abnormalities;
- intestinal obstruction;
- carcinoma;
- idiopathic megacolon;
- drugs – opiates, analgesics, particularly codeine;
- anticholinergic agents;
- diuretics;
- aluminium-containing antacids;
- psychiatric conditions – depression and dementia.

It is easy to see why older people in care homes are vulnerable to constipation and why it warrants the special attention of the registered nurse.

Assessment

The past history of bowel habits should be noted along with any recent changes or difficulties. Any pain on defaecation and the form and consistency of the stool should be included in the assessment. Discussions and observation are valuable in assessing the extent of the problem.

A physical examination should be carried out by a registered nurse, including a rectal examination to detect the presence and consistency of stool in the rectum. The help of the doctor should be sought in order to exclude any abnormalities and to undertake a review of medication.

Planning care depends on the information found on assessment and may include the instigation of a regular regime for the resident, depending on observed behaviour. It is important that the desire to defaecate is responded to quickly or it will pass. This will result in further absorption of water leading to a harder stool and constipation. Time and privacy in the toilet, feeling safe and warm all help towards a normal bowel action.

Fluid and diet play an important role in good bowel management. Studies have demonstrated an association between high dietary fibre intake and colonic faecal loading in immobile older people, (Donald, Smith, Cruikshank et al., 1985). It would, therefore, be inadvisable to increase fibre intake by a large amount, but to offer a varied diet. Barrett (1992) recommends the use of a laxative, depending on the characteristics of the stool and the resident's ability to defaecate.

Laxatives affect bowel action in very different ways and must be used following individual assessment in consultation with the doctor. Initial care should focus on emptying the bowel by suppositories or enema. Barrett (1992) suggests phosphate enemas are most commonly used but suppositories or micro enemas are also helpful.

An osmotic laxative for example Lactulose should be given for those with a hard stool. It increases faecal weight, volume, water and bowel movements and acts within two days. For those with a soft stool, a stimulant laxative is required, such as Senokot, sodium picosulphate, or bisacodyl. Even if older people are given regular laxatives, regular emptying of the lower bowel using an enema or suppositories may still be necessary.

Faecal incontinence is almost always caused by faecal impaction with spurious diarrhoea leaking around the impacted stool and a subsequent gaping anus. If, following a careful assessment by nursing and medical staff the problem is not resolved, then further medical investigations may be indicated.

A planned bowel programme may be used for older people who may not be aware of the need to defaecate. A constipating drug such as codeine phosphate may be used with the use of an enema twice or three times a week to stimulate defaecation. Alternatively, oral medication such as picolax, a potent laxative can be used but should only be used with extreme care and attention.

Promotion of continence in the care setting

Individual assessment of an individual with bladder and/or bowel problems is, of course, crucially important in regaining continence, but equally important is the attitude of staff and residents towards continence. Continence is the normal, healthy state and anything other than that should be noted and addressed immediately. It is always hard to create a balance between physical and emotional or social care. Historically nurses have been criticised for giving less attention to the social and emotional needs of clients. Individualised approaches to care, an examination of ritualistic practices and a genuine desire to reflect the needs and wants of residents will go some way to redressing the balance.

Some general principles which will help are outlined below:

Environment

Private, light, warm and comfortable toilets which are clean and easy to find and access will promote their use, as will environmental clues as to their location for orientation purposes.

Fluid intake

Many incontinent people, and indeed those who care for them, will restrict fluid intake in the mistaken belief that it will help prevent incontinent episodes. In fact, the reverse is true. Older people tend to restrict their fluids to a dangerous level in order to try and avoid incontinence. This may cause electrolyte imbalance, dehydration, malaise, constipation and confusion. Concentrated urine will occur, which is thought to irritate the bladder, giving rise to even more severe urgency and urge incontinence. Therefore an older person should be encouraged to drink about two litres per day. A variety of drinks may be offered and more able residents might be encouraged to help themselves from a tray of drinks placed in the lounge area. It is worth remembering that caffeine is a diuretic which stimulates micturition (Creighton and Stanton, 1990) and so drinking only tea and coffee may not be helpful in promoting continence. The type of drinks and their amount taken later in the evening may well be worth considering.

Care at night

Nocturia and night time incontinence have been mentioned as a common problem among older people. How to resolve the problem is difficult. People have strong opinions about whether to wake residents and help them use the toilet. It can be expected that an older person's bladder will need emptying at least once a night and therefore it could be argued that waking them to use the toilet is encouraging the normal. Older people tend not to sleep as long as younger people during the night. No-one one can be expected to go 12 hours or more without visiting the toilet, and so, if a resident goes to bed before, say 10.30 pm, then either getting up again to use the toilet is necessary, or incontinence will occur. By the same token, if the resident stays in bed late in the morning, then a visit to the toilet, or the use of a commode may be helpful at around 6 am.

Movement and posture

Mobility and good posture will aid a normal diuresis (see Chapter 13).

Food

A varied and interesting diet will encourage the resident to eat well. The likes and dislikes of the resident should be discussed with them and their families if possible. The dietary needs of people from other ethnic and cultural backgrounds should be considered in detail (see Chapter 2).

Staff development

Education programmes may be set up for all members of staff. The local continence advisor may be contacted to find out what courses and study days are available and if he or she may be able of offer training sessions in the home. Most areas have a continence advisor, usually employed by the Community Trust. If you have difficulty locating him or her, contact either the Royal College of Nursing, Continence Care Forum or the Continence Foundation and they will help you locate your specialist. The UKCC (1994) recommends that all staff in nursing homes should attend regular in-service training and have access to relevant external courses.

Aids and appliances

Incontinence will profoundly affect the sufferer's self-esteem and body image. They may worry about possble stains on clothing, or smells of urine and will feel less attractive, avoiding social contact.

If an aid or appliance is to be used, the resident should be involved in the choice of the product they use and the choice (see Chapter 6) should be seen as part of continence promotion strategies. A suitable aid or appliance may be used during the assessment phase to restore confidence or as a permanent measure to manage intractable incontinence. It is crucial to try and help men and women maintain their sexuality. Pads may be seen as 'female products', resembling sanitary wear. They are also likely to be viewed as infantile nappies. Staff who refer to such products as 'nappies' will promote this image amongst the residents.

Toilet substitutes

Four types are commonly used. Commodes for the bedside or for wheeling into toilet areas, over-toilet chairs, urinals for men and women and raised toilet seats. The criteria for the use of commodes and urinals should reflect the ability and choice of the older person. The toilet may be too far for them to reach by walking but this should not prevent the staff from helping individuals to the toilet, perhaps in a wheelchair. Those residents who are mobile may choose or be encouraged to walk back from the toilet (i.e. after the need to urinate or defaecate has been responded to and is no longer the priority in the resident's mind).

Protective pads and pants

There are many disposable plastic-backed pads available. These may be rectangular or shaped and vary in size from small pads for those with stress incontinence to pads which will allow a heavily incontinent resident to sleep undisturbed all night. Many of these pads appear thinner now than a year or so ago because they contain a mix of fluff-pulp and super-absorbent granules. These granules will absorb many times their own weight of moisture.

Stretch pants are part of the same system. They are designed to hold the pad close to the body, so preventing leakage.

The choice can be made according to assessment, so that, for example, large patients with slight leakage can be offered large sized stretch pants and small pads, and a small person with heavy incontinence the opposite.

Some pads are fixed with sticky tapes on the plastic backing and come in various sizes. They may also contain fluff-pulp and super-absorbers. They are not nearly so flexible in that the choice of size (usually 3), depends on the size of the individual. It does not account for the degree of incontinence in the same way as pad and pants systems. Their use will profoundly affect the self-esteem of a resident, and they may feel they are being treated like a baby. Although the product may help the nursing staff, using such a product may not be in the best interests of the resident. They will probably not be able to remove the pad to use toilet facilities themselves and have therefore lost complete control of their bodily functions.

Some companies also offer a 'super' product for night time use. This type of product is usually considerably more expensive and is useful for the management of severe incontinence in older people who may be entirely immobile and where there is no hope of a return to continence. It is always worth looking at several different ranges of products from different companies in order to compare the effectiveness of different products. Additional, back-up services vary from different companies; for example, training sessions for staff and literature to enhance the use of the products. All this should be taken into consideration when deciding which gives best value for money.

Reusable underpads

Again, several companies market underpads, to be used in the bed. They vary in price and the costs of laundering and drying have to be considered. They are designed to be used for patients who do not wear nightwear below the waist, because wet nightwear may well put the resident at great risk of deteriorating skin condition. These under pads protect only the bed.

Male appliances

Simple devices may be extremely useful, such as a non-spill adapter for a bottle. Incontinent men may choose to use a urine collecting system such as a sheath and drainage bag. There are several systems available on prescription, including different sizes, methods of application and methods of adhesion. However, all those available at present on prescription are made of latex and careful observation for adverse skin reactions is needed, particularly when a man first starts using the device. Correct sizing is important or problems such as friction or ischaemia may occur. Men with outflow obstruction should not use this method of management, but should use an indwelling catheter.

Other collecting devices are available such as drip collectors and pubic pressure appliances. Careful fitting is required to make these work effec-. tively, and the expert advice of an appliance fitter or a continence advisor should be sought.

Catheter care

There is a plethora of literature about catheter care, from which certain principles emerge. First of all, urinary indwelling catheters may be of benefit for specific individuals following careful assessment and diagnosis of their problems. They should only be used as a last resort to manage incontinence (Roe, 1992), but may have to be used to relieve bladder outlet obstruction either temporarily prior to surgery, or permanently for those who cannot have surgery. They may also have to be used for people with other voiding disorders. The choice of catheter should be made by considering the length of time the patient is likely to be catheterised and any history of catheter-related problems.

Foley catheters are made in a variety of materials and sizes. Catheters for short-term use, that is those recommended by the manufacturers for up to fourteen days, are made of latex. The advantages are that they are cheap and soft but are prone to encrustation. Latex absorbs water and body moisture causing swelling of the catheter, thereby decreasing the internal diameter (drainage channel) and increasing the external channel (Ryan-Wooley, 1987).

Teflon-coated latex catheters minimise trauma and encrustation to some extent and are recommended by manufacturers to be used for up to four weeks.

Long-term catheters including silicone elastomer-coated latex, hydrogel coated latex or pure silicone are recommended for use up to twelve weeks. They have a smoother surface, minimising trauma, urethral irritation and encrustation (Kunin, Chin and Chambers, 1987).

Catheter sizes

Catheters are available in sizes 8–28 charriere. The French term is used and is equal to about three times the external diameter, measured in millimetres. However, the larger sizes were only ever intended for use following bladder or other urological surgery. For drainage of normal urine, a size 12 or 14 charriere may be used, as these have been found to transport the normal volume of urine excreted by an adult. Larger sizes of catheters have been found to cause leakage (Kennedy, Brocklehurst and Lye 1983) and discomfort (Roe and Brocklehurst, 1987). The urethra is elliptical in shape; it is not a round hole to be filled, and therefore the smaller the size of the catheter, the smaller the disturbance to the natural state there will be and the less leakage round it.

Catheters are manufactured in female and male lengths. Female length catheters are more suitable for some women, so avoiding extra tubing and therefore pooling of urine. The balloon sizes vary from 5–30 ml. Again, the larger size 20–30 ml sizes were only ever intended for use post-operatively and have no place in long-term catheterisation. They cause bladder spasm and leakage of urine (Roe and Brocklehurst, 1987).

All information relating to each catheterisation, including size, balloon size, material and manufacturer's batch number should be recorded in the patient's records.

Drainage bags

There are many urine drainage bags available, with varying capacity, length of inlet tubes and drainage taps. Leg bags are made with a variety of suspension systems suitable for men or women. Two-litre drainage bags may then be attached to the drainage tap of the leg bag for overnight use and then discarded in the morning.

Choosing the right system depends on each patient's needs, remembering that urine must always drain down from the bladder, and the closed system must be maintained.

Care of the catheterised resident

Catheterisation must, of course, be carried out using an aseptic technique, and the use of lubricating, anaesthetic gel has been found to reduce urethral trauma (De Courcy Ireland, 1993).

The benefits of meatal cleansing are doubtful and in a review, Roe (1992) concluded that the use of soap and water with a clean wash cloth, during a daily bath or shower is recommended practice.

Catheters often block, causing retention and leakage. The problem may be twisting or kinking of any part of the tubing, or constipation. However, some patients produce encrustation from mineral salts. Getcliffe (1993) found that the regular use of a small amount (10–20 ml) of Suby G or mandelic acid as a bladder washout reduced encrustation. Leakage may also be caused by the use of too large a catheter allowing urine to pass round the catheter. It would, therefore, be advantageous to reduce the size when changing the catheter. If leakage continues even when using a size 12 or 14, and urine is also draining well (i.e. there does not appear to be any blockage) then a small dose of an anticholinergic drug may be indicated to reduce detrusor contractions.

Conclusion

The nurse's attitude towards the promotion of urinary and faecal continence is a crucial and often under-estimated aspect of effective and quality care for older people. Incontinence of both urine and faeces is a symptom and requires assessment and investigation to assist in either the resolution or minimisation of the problem. A great deterrent to successful intervention in continence promotion is inconstancy in the implementation of planned strategies and unrealistic expectations of rapid and sometimes full recovery. Promotion of continence and the management of incontinence is complex. It demands knowledge and skills which should be within the realms of all registered nurses. Specialist help, advice and expert knowledge is available through the continence advisor and guidance on health authorities' responsibilities for the provision of such services (NHSE, 1995) should facilitate access to this expertise. The Continence Foundation and the Royal College of Nursing Continence Care Forum can both be a source of information and advice. Helping individuals with their need to eliminate either urine or faeces is an integral part of nursing. Nurses have a responsibility to assess and plan for the restoration of continence where this is achievable and to actively seek to minimise the situation where continence is an unresolvable chronic challenge. To achieve this successfully the nurse will act with compassionate sensitivity. Wells(1992) described the use of pads as helpful 'wetting' management but not as a solution to incontinence. The promotion of continence is dependent on creative and dynamic intervention from nurses who have the requisite knowledge, skills and motivation.

Useful contacts

The Continence Foundation, 2 Doughty Street, London WC1N 2PH.
The Continence Care Forum, Royal College of Nursing, 20 Cavendish Square, London W1M 0B.

References

Barrett, J.A. (1992) Faecal Incontinence. In B. H. Roe (ed.) *Clinical Nursing Practice; The Promotion and Management of Continence.* Prentice Hall International (UK) Ltd.

Brink, C.A., Sampselle, C.M., Wells, T.J. et al. (1989) A digital test for pelvic muscle strength in older women with urinary incontinence. *Nursing Research,* **38**(4), 196–199.

Burgio, L.D., McCormick, K.A., Scheve, A.S. et al. (1994) The effects of changing prompted voiding schedules in the treatment of incontinence in nursing home residents. *Journal of the American Geriatrics Society,* **42** (3), 315–320.

Creighton, S. and Stanton, S. (1990) Caffeine: does it affect your bladder? *British Journal of Urology,* **66**, 613–614.

De Courcy Ireland, K. (1993) An issue of sensitivity — use of anaesthetic gel in catheterising women. *Professional Nurse,* August.

Department of Health (1992a) Health and Personal Social Services Statistics for England. London: HMSO.

Department of Health (1992b) An Agenda for Action for Continence Services. London: HMSO.

Donald, L.P., Smith, R.G., Cruikshank, J.G. et al. (1985) A study of constipation in the elderly living at home. *Gerontology*, **3**, 1, 112–115.

Duffin, H.M. (1992) Assessment of Urinary Incontinence. In B.H. Roe (ed.) *Clinical Nursing Practice: The Promotion and Management of Continence.* Prentice Hall International (UK) Ltd.

Ebersole, P. and Hess, P. (1990) Toward Healthy Aging: human needs and nursing response. The C.V. Mosby Company.

Getcliffe, K. (1993) Freeing the System. *Nursing Standard*, **8**, 7, 16–18.

Jilek, R. (1993) Elderly toileting: is two hourly too often? *Nursing Standard*, **7**, 47, 25–26.

Jirovec, M.M. and Thelma Wells, T.J. (1990) Urinary Incontinence in Nursing Home Residents with Dementia: The Mobility–Cognition Paradigm. *Applied Nursing Research*, **3**, 3 (August) 112–117.

Kennedy, A.P., Brocklehurst, J.C., and Lye, M.D.W. (1983) Factors related to the problems of long term catheterisation. *Journal of Advanced Nursing*, **8** (3), 207–212.

Kunin, C.M., Chin, Q.F. and Chambers S. (1987) Formation of encrustations on indwelling urinary catheters in the eldery: a comparison of different types of catheter materials in blockers and non-blockers. *The Journal of Urology*, **138**, 809–902.

Laycock, J. (1992) Pelvic floor education for the promotion of contintence. In B.H. Roe (ed.) *Clinical Nursing: The Promotion and Management of Continence*. Prentice Hall International (UK) Ltd.

McClymont, M., Thomas, S. and Denham, M. (1991) *Health visiting and elderly people: a health promotion challenge*. Churchill Livingstone.

Moody, H. (1990) *Incontinence: patient problems and nursing care*. Heinemann.

National Health Service Executive (1995) *Health Authorities Responsibilities for the Provision of Continuing Care*. London: HMSO.

Norton, C. (1986) *Nursing for Continence*. Bucks: Beaconsfield Ltd.

O'Brien, J., Austin, M., Sethi, P. and O'Boyle, P. (1991) Urinary Incontinence Prevalence, need for treatment, and effectiveness of intervention by nurse. *British Medical Journal*, **303**, 1308–1312.

Ouslander, J., Morishita, B., Blaustein, J. et al. (1987) Clinical, functional and psychosocial characteristics of an incontinent nursing home population. *Journal of Gerontology*, **42**, 631.

Ouslander, J., Schnelle, J., Simmons, S. Bates-Jensen, B. and Zeitlin, M. (1993) The dark side of incontinence: Night time incontinence in nursing home residents. *Journal of the American Geriatrics Society*, **41**, 371–376.

Palmer, M.H. (1991) Risk Factors for Urinary Incontinence one year after Nursing Home Admission. *Research in Nursing and Health*, **14**, 6, 405.

Resnick, N. (1990) Non-invasive diagnosis of the patient with complex incontinence. *International Journal of Experiments and Clinical Gerontology*, **8**(18) 12.

Roe, B.H. (1992) *Clinical Nursing Practice: The Promotion and Management of Continence*. Prentice Hall International (UK) Ltd.

Roe, B.H. and Brocklehurst, J.C. (1987) Study of Patients with indwelling catheters. *Journal of Advanced Nursing*, **12**, 713–718.

Rowe, J. (1988) Renal System. In J. Rowe and R. Besdine (eds.) *Geriactric Medicine* (2nd edition). Little, Brown and Co.

Ryan-Wooley, B. (1987) Aids for the Management of Incontinence. King's Fund.

UKCC (1994) Professional Conduct – Occasional Report on Standards of Nursing in Nursing Homes. United Kingdom Central Council for Nursing, Midwifery and Health Visiting.

Wells, T. (1992) Foreword, in Roe B.H. *Clinical Nursing Practice: The Promotion and Management of Continence.* Prentice Hall International (UK) Ltd.

Whippo, C.C. and Crason, N.S. (1989) Bacteriuria and urinary incontinence in aged female nursing home residents. *Journal of Advanced Nursing*, **14**, 217–225.

15

Wound Care

Mary Clay

Introduction

Wound care may be an important aspect of nurses' work with older people in care homes, and nurses need a sound understanding of the subject in order that appropriate treatments can be given. In addition to being a problem for patients and care staff, wounds are an enormous drain on financial resources. There appear to be no figures on the cost of wounds or pressure sores in care homes. However, the estimated annual NHS costs of wound care for older people are in the region of £950 million (Lewis, 1994). Treating pressure sores in the UK costs between £150 and £200 million annually (Morison, 1990a). For one patient only, in 1987, the total costs were calculated to be almost £26 000 (Fletcher, 1994). Leg ulcers are similarly expensive, the expenditure per patient per annum being around £1 000–£5 200. In 1989 the total NHS treatment costs for venous leg ulcers were between £300 and £600 million (Wilson, 1989). In addition, litigation is a cost not often considered. One patient who developed a pressure sore was awarded £100 000 (Bridel, 1992). It is immediately clear therefore that wound care impacts on health, quality of life, and resources.

Since wound management has altered dramatically over the last twenty years, nurses are now presented with a bewildering choice of treatments. Under the Scope of Professional Practice (UKCC, 1992b), nurses need to continuously review wound management practices, and select only those treatments which are supported by published research and objective clinical evaluation (Flannagan, 1994). In fact, researchers often express frustration that their findings are not implemented in clinical practice (Altmeyer, 1993). Linking our practice to the UKCC Scope of Professional Practice (UKCC, 1992b), and Code of Professional Conduct (UKCC, 1992a) may assist with this.

According to Young (1990), one of the great unmet needs in wound care is 'the provision of very basic information by reliable and simple means'. He points out that, while the glamour may lie at the cutting edge of technology, the greatest need is for more widepsread implementation of simple techniques, a thorough knowledge of which he feels are lacking.

This chapter attempts to redress this balance.

Definitions

The most common wounds in care homes are pressure sores, leg ulcers and wounds resulting from minor trauma. The only published survey specific to nursing homes found that 80 per cent of homes were treating either surgical wounds (open or closed), fungating wounds, or delayed primary suturing. The numbers of homes treating pressure sores and leg ulcers were approximately equal.

A **wound** can be defined as 'the loss of continuity of skin, causing disruption of the normal tissue pattern' (Ayton, 1985). Whether the wounds are abrasions, cuts, burns, or ulcers, the same biochemical and cellular processes are involved in healing (Morison, 1994).

A **pressure sore** is 'a localised area of tissue necrosis that usually occurs over a bony prominence. It is assessed as having been caused primarily by unrelieved pressure, shearing, friction or a combination of these forces' (Reid and Morison, 1994). Pressure sores are also known as decubitus ulcers, bed sores and pressure ulcers (Collier, 1994). Pressure sores begin to develop when pressure on local blood vessels causes them to become blocked with erythrocytes, and the endothelial cells swell. As a result, ischaemia or thrombosis occurs, leading to tissue necrosis. (Lester, 1992).

A **leg ulcer** is a 'tissue breakdown of the leg or foot due to any cause' (Cullum, 1994).

Traumatic wounds are those 'caused by injury, e.g. burns and lacerations' (University of Dundee, 1993).

Wound healing

A wound is usually considered to have healed when it has been resurfaced with epithelium and it looks pink, smooth and dry. However, it is still vulnerable to trauma, and healing actually continues for some months until skin regains most of its strength.

Primary healing (from a clean cut, closed by sutures, needing little new tissue) tends to be rapid.

Secondary healing (involving deeper layers of tissue loss) tends to vary between weeks and months. In exceptional cases, healing may never be achieved. Secondary healing is likely to be prevalent in most nursing homes.

Healing has three overlapping phases – inflammation, proliferation, and maturation.

Inflammation is the first response to healing. It activates protective mechanisms, the signs of which are heat, redness, pain, swelling and loss of function. Inflammation occurs through chemicals which cause blood vessel dilatation, increased capillary permeability, oedema and stimulation of pain fibres. This normal phase of healing may be lengthy in traumatic wounds with widespread damage. If inflammation is intensified and prolonged, this may indicate infection or harmful topical agents. Due to the increased capillary permeability, protein-rich fluid leaks into the tissues. This inflammatory exudate forms on the wound surface, and will be most marked when the tissues are oedematous, or the inflammation is intense. Exudate forms an important part of the wound's defence system as it contains proteins, including antibodies. It is suggested that there are growth-promoting substances in exudate, which are particularly beneficial in healing chronic wounds, and that the exudate should therefore be kept in contact with the wound by occlusive dressings. Enzymes are released, which digest dead tissue (a process known as autolysis). As healing progresses the amount of exudate decreases until the wound is covered by epithelial tissue.

The body's defences, for example the immune system, influence the healing process. The principal cells in the immune response are lymphocytes, monocytes and macrophages. Therefore a compromised immune system will delay healing, for example in patients who are taking immune-suppressive drugs, are HIV positive, or have other chronic infections.

Proliferation is a repairing phase in wound healing. Cells called macrophages are attracted to the wound site. These combine with oxygen and other factors to promote capillary growth and the production of collagen. This, in turn, leads to the formation of granulation tissue.

Granulation occurs in the transition phase between inflammation and repair. It leads to the formation of new blood vessels (angiogenesis). Granulation tissue is red, moist and fragile connective tissue that fills in the wound during proliferation. This process normally begins a few days after injury.

Epithelialisation is the process whereby the wound is resurfaced with new epithelium. Initially attachment of the new surface to underlying tissue is fragile, and can be easily disrupted. The epithelialisation rate may be enhanced by a moist local environment. Temperature variation, infection and changes in the bodily acidity may cause delays in tissue granulation, and hence epithelialisation.

Maturation is the final stage of wound healing, when collagen is converted and reorganised. Cellular activity and blood supply reduce. Dermal healing forms scar tissue which initially looks flat, then becomes red, firm and raised. Finally the scar fades, softens and becomes flatter (University of Dundee, 1993).

Wound healing in older people

Ageing skin

Age-related skin changes affect both older people's susceptibility to wounds, and the wound healing process.

Epidermal cell renewal time increases by one-third after 50 years of age. Because of this, slower replacement of epidermal cells, wound healing is approximately 50 per cent slower than at 35 years of age. Ageing decreases the inflammatory response. Collagen reduction also occurs with ageing, and this affects wound healing in that the skin is less able to stretch and thus more likely to tear.

The dermis becomes thinner in the absence of subcutaneous fat. The aged skin loses resilience and moisture, and takes on a characteristic dryness. The loss of elasticity affects blood vessels, particularly the arteries. Elastic fibres fray, split, straighten and fragment. Calcium which leaves the bone is deposited in the vessels.

These age-related changes decrease the lumen of vessels, and cause the blood flow to various organs to become uneven. Peripheral resistance in the vessels increases as a consequence of the calcium deposits and reduced elasticity. The layers in the skin are then thinner and more fragile. The cell turnover in older skin is reduced and healing is delayed.

In spite of slower healing, older people's wounds can heal satisfactorily, and often with a good cosmetic result.

Factors influencing wound healing in older people.

A number of other factors also influence wound healing in older people. These include:

Adverse local conditions at the wound site: for example, recurrent trauma, foreign bodies, dehydration, excess exudate, oedema, necrotic tissue, infection, excess metabolic waste products, vascular insufficiency, local hypoxia, and fall in wound temperature.

Adverse effects of other therapies: for example, cytotoxic drugs, prolonged use of high-dose steroids, and radiation therapy.

Poor nutrition, or anaemia: an older person's protein and calorie requirements are likely to be higher when wounds are healing. Sufficient intake and absorption of vitamins such as A and C, and minerals such as zinc and iron, are also required for optimum healing. (Vitamin C is essential for collagen regeneration.)

Respiratory and cardiovascular disorders: may cause reduced blood supply to a wound. This is likely to have a significant effect on wound healing as the growing edge of a wound is an area of high metabolic activity. Hypoxia (lack of oxygen) at the wound edge not only inhibits the production of epithelial cells, fibroblasts and collagen, but also the ability of macrophages to destroy bacteria.

Immune disorders: may cause decreased resistance to infection.

Endocrine and metabolic disorders: wounds may be slower to heal if the underlying condition is unstable. This is particularly so with diabetic ulcers, where there is an added complication of peripheral vascular disease.

Concurrent health problems: these include immobility, sensory impairments, or even altered consciousness can directly or indirectly affect wound healing. One of the most common concurrent problems in care homes is incontinence. There is a high correlation between incontinence and pressure sores, as urine can cause maceration (sogginess) and excoriation (soreness) of the skin, making it more vulnerable to superficial abrasion.

Inappropriate wound management: failure to identify and correct the underlying cause of the wound, the application of inappropriate topical agents and primary wound dressings, or poor dressing technique can all delay healing (Morison, 1994).

Psychosocial factors: these are also likely to affect older people; for example loss of motivation, multiple life changes, bereavement, altered body image resulting in actual or perceived problems with social relationships, lack of belief in the effectiveness of treatment, or negative attitudes of staff to treatments or healing, will all have an impact (Morison, 1994).

Prevention of wounds

Pressure sores

Virtually all pressure sores are primarily due to unrelieved pressure, and most usually occur in relatively or totally immobile patients where the skin and the underlying tissues are directly compressed between the bone and another hard surface, such as a bed or a chair. The most common sites for pressure sore development are the sacrum, trochanters of the femurs (in the hip joints), ischial tuberosities (sitting bones), and heels. There is broad agreement that most pressure sores could be prevented, if an active prevention plan is implemented (Bridel, 1992).

The relief of pressure is the key to prevention. This can be achieved by regular changes in position, and by the use of pressure-relieving devices, such as heel protectors, cushions, mattresses and beds. Good nutrition and adequate hydration are the second most important factors. The effective management of incontinence, where continence cannot be achieved, is also of great importance (see Chapter 13).

Morison (1994) suggests the use of a ten-point action plan for the prevention and management of pressure sores (see Table 15.1).

Table 15.1:   *Preventing and managing pressure sores – Morison's ten point action plan*

1. Assess the risk of pressure sore development within two hours of admission, using a reliable and valid tool (such as Norton (1962), or Waterlow (1988)).
2. Reassess the risk whenever there is a material change in the patient's condition.
3. Use a patient support system appropriate to the patient's risk score within two hours of admission.
4. Devise a mobility/turning schedule appropriate to the patient's risk and chart position changes. (The aim is to keep the patient off broken skin and high-risk sites as much as possible, bearing in mind the need for rest, meals and visiting).

5. Inspect high-risk sites whenever re-positioning; reassess pressure sores daily; chart treatment and healing.
6. Maintain skin integrity (for example by always cleansing after urine or faeces have been on the skin, not rubbing the skin and not using excess soap).
7. With the aid of a dietitian, assess the patient's nutritional status and any special dietary requirements. Keep the patient well hydrated.
8. Alleviate the effects of other concurrent debilitating conditions where possible.
9. Identify and attempt to correct any problems associated with sleep.
10. Remember the importance of psychological support.

A wide variety of pressure-relieving devices, made by different manufacturers, are currently available. These include:

- alternating pressure mattresses and overlays (e.g. Pegasus Airwave System, and Nimbus Dynamic Flotation System);
- water beds (e.g. Beaufort-Winchester);
- air-fluidised beds (e.g. Clinitron);
- low air-loss bed systems (e.g. Medicus);
- low pressure air beds (e.g. Simpson-Edinburgh);
- cut foam mattresses (e.g. Polyfloat);
- net suspension beds (e.g. Mecabed);
- silicone fibre overlays (e.g. Spenco and Superdown); and
- a wide range of chair cushions.

Manufacturers are usually willing to demonstrate their products and to produce the results of clinical trials which they have undergone.

Morison (1990a) suggests that ideal support systems should:

- distribute pressure evenly;
- minimise friction and shearing forces;
- provide a comfortable, well ventilated patient/resident support surface;
- allow unrestricted movement;
- be acceptable to the patient/resident;
- allow nursing care to be given unimpeded;
- be easily maintained; and
- be inexpensive.

Leg ulcers

Leg ulcers are difficult to prevent. They tend to be chronic wounds, which form where a predisposing condition impairs both tissue integrity and healing. Common examples are impaired venous damage due to venous hypertension, and impaired arterial blood supply due to peripheral vascular disease. No studies have specifically examined criteria for leg ulcer susceptibility (Cullum, 1994), although ulceration is often preceded by skin changes and pigmentation.

The management of predisposing factors and underlying disease is possibly the most important preventative measure. For example, anyone who has evidence of peripheral vascular disease should be referred for a vascular assessment. Residents with varicose veins should be encouraged to avoid standing or sitting for long, continuous periods. Foot and leg elevation is essential when resting. Particularly important is the activation of the calf muscle pump, which should be achieved by ankle movement and exercise. Residents should be advised to avoid obstructing veins by wearing tight socks, girdles or garters, and to avoid crossing their legs when sitting.

Leg ulcer prevention may be assisted by giving up smoking, eating a well-balanced diet, avoiding obesity, and undertaking suitable exercise, especially if mobility is impaired.

Recent research suggests that 300 mg of enteric-coated aspirin taken daily could speed up the healing of chronic venous leg ulcers (Layton et al., 1994). However this is a small study and the reason for the effect is unknown.

Once a venous ulcer has healed, it is important to prevent recurrence. High-quality, below-knee Class 11 compression stockings are available on drug tariff. Careful ankle and calf measurement are essential to ensure a correct fit, and hosiery should be replaced at three monthly intervals.

Prevention of diabetic foot ulcers

The feet of people with diabetes should be examined regularly in order to identify dry skin calluses, clawed toes, prominent metatarsal heads, bunions, limited joint mobility, or for signs of infection. Regular nail care, and the removal of excess calluses by a qualified chiropodist is essential. The formation of dry skin is to be avoided as it may lead to cracking and contribute to excess callus formation. Extra depth shoes with insoles should be provided and general pressure-reducing management should be applied (Young, 1993).

Prevention of traumatic wounds

While some traumatic wounds can be avoided by accident prevention strategies, many minor injuries are still likely to occur among care home residents, particularly those who are ambulant but frail. If older people in nursing homes are encouraged to be independent, especially if this involves a degree or risk-taking, some minor wounds resulting from knocks or falls are inevitable.

Assessment of wounds

Nurses working in care homes have responsibility for the assessment and management of wounds, and are deemed accountable for both their actions and omissions (UKCC, 1992a). Accurate and ongoing assessment is essential in planning appropriate wound management, and for evaluating its effectiveness.

Wound assessment can benefit from the use of a nursing model. For example, Roper, Logan and Tierney's Activities of Living Model (1980) can be used as the framework for the assessment of the wound, as well as for the individual overall. Using the model helps to highlight the implications of the wound in relation to the everyday life of the patient. It also helps to integrate not only specific treatments, but also other aspects of care such as the management of predisposing factors, the relief of symptoms, and the prevention of further associated problems. All of these factors may contribute to delayed wound healing (Collier, 1994; Bethell, 1994). Thus the wound is not dealt with in isolation, but rather as part of the planned care.

The location of chronic wounds will often indicate their cause, for example, wounds directly above bony prominences are most likely to be pressure ulcers. The site of the leg ulcer will usually indicate whether it is arterial or venous in origin.

Wound pain should be assessed for its type, severity, duration and precipitating factors. Patient history-taking should include questioning about cramping pains in the legs at night, and whether the pain is relieved by lowering the legs over the bedside, as this is frequently an indicator of poor arterial blood supply. It may be difficult for nurses to differentiate objectively between words used by patients to describe their pain. Descriptive, or visual analogue scales, may be helpful (e.g. the McGill Pain Questionnaire (Melzack, 1975)).

It is important to detect whether nerve endings are exposed, and also if the pain increases, reduces or ceases when the dressing is applied, or when the limb is elevated.

Assessment of the patient's cognitive abilities and his or her current level of knowledge of the condition is important so that appropriate patient education can be established.

Wound assessment tools

A simple method of assessing wounds is by their predominant colour, as this not only indicates the physiological status, but also highlights the treatment objective. Flannigan (1990) suggests the following:

- Black wounds: necrotic areas of dehydrated dead tissue which, if not removed, will prolong the healing process and harbour pathogenic organisms.
- Yellow wounds: sloughy, with dead cells and debris in the base of the wound.
- Red wounds: granulating, bright in colour, and moist.
- Pink wounds: epithelialising over granulation tissue.
- Green wounds: infected. Other signs of infection include excessive exudate, copious pus, systematic patient pyrexia, tachycardia and offensive odour.

Other wound assessment tools are more complex. The Open Wounds Assessment Chart by Morison (1994) provides a comprehensive format for the ongoing assessment of wounds. Progress and complications can easily be identified using this documentation, shown in Table 15.2.

Table 15.2: *The Open Wounds Assessment Chart (Morison, 1994)*

Type of wound (pressure sore, fungating carcinoma etc.) ....

Location...

How long has wound been open? ....

General patient factors which may delay healing (e.g. malnutrition, diabetes, other chronic infection) ....

Allergies to wound care products ....

Previous treatments tried (comment on success/problems) ....

Wound factors and date

1. Nature of wound bed					
(tick more than one if appropriate)					
a. healthy granulation					
b. epithelialisation visible					
c. soft slough					
d. hard black/brown necrotic tissue					
e. other					
2. Exudate					
a. colour					
b. type (e.g. purulent)					
c. appropriate amount: marked/moderate/ minimal/none					
3. Odour					
Offensive/some/none					
4. Pain (site)					
a. at wound itself					
b. elsewhere (specify)					
5. Pain (frequency)					
Continuous/intermittent/ only at dressing changes/none					
6. Pain (severity)					
Patient's score (0–10)					
7. Wound margin					
a. erythema					
b. oedematous					
8. General condition of surrounding skin					
(e.g. dry, clammy, wet eczema)					
9. Infection					
a. suspected					
b. wound swab sent					
c. confirmed (specify organism)					

Describing the wound

The size of the wound should be measured initially, and at regular intervals. There are a number of methods of visually assessing wounds, such as computer mapping, polaroid photography, or tracing the wound margin using clean transparent film. The manufacturers of wound dressings (such as Convatec) supply purpose-made graphed film charts free of charge. Although this may be a crude measurement, it does confirm any change in wound size, and is likely to be more valuable than nurses' subjective comments. Photographing wounds at regular intervals has the advantage that visiting doctors can see how the wound is progressing without unnecessarily removing the dressings, and thus disturbing the healing process.

High frequency ultrasound scanning (Miller, 1994a) and video image analysis (Boardman, Melhuish and Harding, 1994), provide more detailed and accurate information for wound assessment, but are not widely available.

Classification of pressure sores

Standardising the classification of pressure sores can help avoid varying and ambiguous descriptions. It can also help facilitate audits of pressure sore care and comparisons between different institutions. It should also make it easier to compare clinical trials of wound dressings and pressure-relieving devices.

Reid and Morison (1994) reviewed UK pressure sore classification systems and, with a panel of experts, drew up a United Kingdom Consensus Classification (see Table 15.3).

Table 15.3:   *The UK Consensus Pressure Sore Classification*

Stage 0:   No clinical evidence of a pressure sore.
- 0.0:   Normal appearance skin intact.
- 0.1:   Healed with scarring.
- 0.2:   Tissue damage, but not assessed as a pressure sore.

Stage 1.   Discolouration of intact skin-light finger pressure applied to the site does not alter the discolouration.
- 1.1:   Non-blanchable erythema with increased local heat.
- 1.2:   Blue/purple/black discolouration. The sore is at least Stage 1.

Stage 2.   Partial thickness skin loss or damage involving epidermis and or dermis.
- 2.1:   Blister.
- 2.2:   Abrasion.
- 2.3:   Shallow ulcer, without undermining of adjacent tissue.
- 2.4:   Any of these with underlying blue/purple/black discolouration or induration. This sore is at least Stage 2.

Stage 3.   Full thickness skin loss involving damage or necrosis of subcutaneous tissue but not extending to underlying bone, tendon or joint capsule.

3.1:   Crater, without undermining of adjacent tissue.
3.2:   Crater, with undermining of adjacent tissue.
3.3:   Sinus, the full extent of which is not certain.
3.4:   Full thickness skin loss, but wound bed covered with necrotic tissue (hard or leathery black/brown or softer tissue or softer yellow/cream/grey slough) which masks the true extent of the tissue damage. The sore is at least Stage 3. (Until debrided it is not possible to observe whether damage extends into muscle or involves damage to bone or supporting structures).

Stage 4.   Full thickness skin loss with extensive destruction and tissue necrosis extending to underlying bone, tendon or capsule.

4.1:   Visible exposure of bone, tendon or joint capsule.
4.2:   Sinus assessed as extending to bone, tendon or capsule.

Third-digit classification for the nature of the wound bed.
x.x0:   Not applicable, intact skin.
x.x1:   Clean, with partial epithelialisation.
x.x2:   Clean, with or without granulation but no obvious epithelialisation.
x.x3:   Soft slough, cream/yellow/green in colour.
x.x4:   Hard or leathery black/brown necrotic (dead/avascular) tissue.

Fourth-digit classification for the infective complications.
x.xx0:   No inflammation surrounding the wound bed.
x.xx1:   Inflammation surrounding the wound bed.
x.xx2:   Cellulitis bacteriologically confirmed.

This classification is easy to follow and depends on visual observation only (except for bacteriological confirmation of infection). The user can choose the degree of precision needed, using either two-, three- or four-digit codes.

Leg ulcers

In addition to a full health assessment, and specific assessment of the wound, patients presenting with leg ulcers should have an assessment of the surrounding skin, as this may help to diagnose the ulcer type. For example, the skin around venous ulcers is liable to be stained and pigmented, with signs of eczema, oedema and ankle flare (caused by dilated small veins around the ankle). In the case of arterial ulceration the skin may be thin, shiny, and hairless due to the malnourishment of the tissues. Toe nails are likely to be thickened and the affected limb cold and pale. Both legs and the skin surrounding the ulcers should be examined for signs of ischaemia.

Anyone presenting with leg ulceration should have their foot pulses checked. If this cannot be recorded (either due to their absence or to oedema) then referral should be made for the measurement of the brachial-to-ankle pressure ratio using the non-invasive Doppler technique. In the case of deep diabetic ulcers, X-rays should form part of assessment.

The inadequate assessment of leg ulcers can lead to inadequate or hazardous treatment regimes (Moffat, 1994). For example compression therapy can be disastrous if applied to an ischaemic limb.

Wagner (1981) devised a classification system for vascular ulcers (see Table 15.4).

Table 15.4:   *Classification of leg ulcers (Wagner, 1981)*

Grade 1:   Superficial ulcers.
Grade 2:   Deep ulcer with underlying tendon involvement.
Grade 3:   Deep ulcer with bone involvement causing osteomyelitis.
Grade 4:   Localised gangrene which commonly occurs at the end of the toes and heels.
Grade 5:   Extensive gangrene, extensive necrosis of the foot due to arterial occlusion.

Treatment of wounds

In order for wound care in nursing homes to be carried out systematically, Moody (1993) suggests that protocols should be developed. Protocols should be based on current knowledge, but evaluated periodically and updated in the light of new research, changing practices and new products.

The general principles of management are:

- to remove the extrinsic factors which delay healing such as unrelieved pressure, shearing and frictional forces,
- to alleviate the effects of the intrinsic factors which contribute to tissue breakdown, such as malnutrition, incontinence and recurrent illness; and
- to provide the optimum local environment for healing at the wound site (Morison, 1990a).

The large variety of dressings now available can make the task of choosing the optimum dressing a confusing experience. An understanding of the concept of the ideal wound-healing environment, however, will give nurses a logical basis for dressing selection (Miller, 1994b).

It is important that nurses follow appropriate protocols. In one study, it was found that inappropriate dressings were being used in approximately 85 per cent of cases (Murray, 1988).

The United Kingdom Drug Tariff limits the availability of some drugs and dressings for use in the community on NHS prescription. There may therefore be occasions when the dressing which is considered the most appropriate may not be available in care homes, and the regime may have to be changed on discharge from hospital, solely for this reason. This is not to be recommended as it may inhibit the healing process. Items suggested by Morgan (1992a) as useful suitable additions to the Drug Tariff include hydrocolloid paste for cavity wounds, alginate packing/ribbon for cavity wounds and a deodorising dressing. These can sometimes be obtained directly from the manufacturers.

Characteristics of the ideal wound dressing

An ideal wound dressing could be defined as 'a material which, when applied to the surface of a wound, provides and maintains an environment in which healing can take place at the maximum rate' (Turner, Schmidt and Harding, 1986). The ideal wound dressing therefore maintains a moist environment at the wound site, while removing excess exudate and toxic compounds.

Dressings which promote a **moist environment** or which maintain tissue hydration are referred to as occlusive dressings. Examples of this type of dressings are hydrocolloids, alginates, vapour-permeable films, hydrogels and foam dressings.

An ideal dressing provides **thermal insulation** is **impermeable to bacteria**, is **non-toxic** and **non-allergenic**.

It is **non-adherent** and causes **minimal trauma** to the wound on removal.

It is **comfortable** and conformable to awkward sites, provides protection from mechanical trauma and requires infrequent dressing changes (Morison, 1994). A suitable dressing provides **warmth**. Foam and hydrocolloid dressings will maintain wound temperatures at 35°C whereas, with gauze dressings, wound temperature would be 8° lower. Wound temperature is important as it has been found that cellular activity slows down when wound temperature decreases. One study found that it took 40 minutes for wounds to regain their original temperature and three hours for normal cellular activity to be resumed after wound cleansing.

Researchers have found that wounds heal more effectively and that infection is reduced in a **slightly acid** environment (Tsukada, Tokunaja, Iwana, et al., 1992). Hydrocolloid dressings have been shown to produce a wound pH of between 5.6 and 6.7, whereas vapour-permeable film dressings create a pH of around 7.1 (Varghese, Arthur, Canter and Callweed, 1986). Although further research is required it would appear that wound healing accelerates in a slightly acid environment.

Angiogenesis (the formation of new vessels) has been found to take place rapidly in the **hypoxic** environment created by hydrocolloid dressings (Cherry and Ryan, 1985). Miller (1994b) therefore suggests the use of hydrocolloid dressings for granulating wounds and oxygen-permeable dressings for epithelialising wounds. On the other hand, outstanding results have been reported by the use of hyperbaric oxygen in non-healing wounds (Heng, Pilgrim and Beck, 1984).

Treatments not recommended

- Continual washing with soap and water is discouraged as it may affect the skin's normal pH and remove natural oils.
- The use of massage can impair the blood circulation to a potential pressure area, and macerate the underlying tissue.
- The use of sorbo rings can make a sacral pressure sore worse by creating a tourniquet effect and occluding the microcirculation (Pudner, 1994).

Although these practices have not been advocated in the United Kingdom for many years they are still in use.

The use of raw eggs was once a popular treatment for pressure sores but has been specifically prohibited by the Department of Health since 1988 (Ref.: EL (88) CO/10).

Gentian violet was once used for its antibacterial properties, and as an astringent to dry up macerated skin, for example around an ulcer, but this has also been withdrawn from use in open wounds. Manufacturers were advised of this in 1987 when the substance was found to be carcinogenic in animals.

Gauze or other dry dressings are not advocated as they do not create the right environment to promote healing. Cotton wool, which is often used to cleanse wounds, sheds fibres into the wound and these can become the focus for bacteria and lead to infection (Johnson, 1988).

Gauze packing is not recommended as the unequal pressures exerted on the wound bed disrupt the micro-circulation and thereby delay wound healing.

Hypochlorites, for example eusol, hydrogen peroxide and milton should not be used. They interfere with collagen synthesis, damage epithelial cells, damage microcirculation and attack cell walls of coliform organisms thus producing endotoxins, which, when absorbed, give rise to varying degrees of renal failure (Morison, 1990b). The dangers of eusol and hypochlorites, although they are well documented may need to be explained especially to medical staff who have prescribed them successfully in the past, and who may be unaware that there are now safer alternatives available. (It may be appropriate to refer them to research studies, for example, Brennan and Leaper (1985), Brennan, Foster and Leaper (1986), Leaper and Simpson (1986).)

Topical antibiotics, may cause skin sensitivity and reactions, and encourage resistant strains of bacteria. Although prescribable, sofra-tulle, fucidin intertulle and cicatrin are not recommended for wound care for the these reasons (Morgan, 1992a).

Oxygen given topically was once a popular treatment, but it dries out the wound thereby preventing a moist wound which is the desired environment to promote healing. It also affects tissue perfusion (Royal Marsden Hospital, 1990).

Disinfectants, for example chlorhexidine and povidone iodine are not recommended. Disinfectant solutions kill fibroblasts and therefore hamper the natural repair process (Bloomsbury and Islington Health Authority, 1991).

Wound cleansing

The aim of wound cleansing is to help create the optimum conditions for wound healing prior to the application of a wound dressing. Wound cleansing therefore involves the removal of debris, which may include foreign material, devitalised (i.e. dead or ischaemic) soft tissue, excess slough, necrotic tissue, loose debris and stale exudate, bacteria and micro-organisms whose continued presence might delay healing and act as a focus for infection.

The recommended solution is normal saline (0.9 per cent sodium chloride) sterile solution for all wound cleansing. It has the advantage of being non-toxic and has no adverse effect on healing. Each wound should be assessed and only cleansed when necessary. If a wound is grossly contaminated, wound cleansing is necessary at every dressing change to prevent delayed healing. On the other hand if the wound is clean and there is little exudate and it is healthily granulating, then repeated cleaning may do more harm than good, by traumatising newly produced and delicate tissues, by reducing the surface temperature of the wound and by removing exudate which itself may have bacteridical properties. The solution should be as close to body temperature as possible. Irrigation should be used in preference to wiping, since there is a risk of contaminating the wound or removing epithelialising cells (Morison, 1990b).

Normal saline is now available in a multi-use aerosol and a research study by Lawerence, Lilly and Kidson (1994) has found it to be an appropriate product for wound irrigation. A chronic wound may be cleansed by soaking in a bath or shower although this may be unacceptable to the cultures of some ethnic groups.

The range of wound management products

The variety of wound management products is extensive. Some examples are:

● Calcium alginates (absorbent haemostatic dressings derived from seaweed, which form a viscous gel over the wound surface, e.g. Kaltostat* and Sorbsan*).
● De-odourisers (dressings which contain activated charcoal to absorb odours for example in fungating carcinomas, e.g. Metrop*, Actisorb and Kaltocarb).
● Enzymes (proteins which will catalyse a biological reaction, e.g. Varidase*).
● Hydrocolloids (dressings containing a colloid system in which water is a dispersion medium. Normally available as wafers, e.g. Granuflex*, Comfeel* and Tagasorb*).

- Hydrogels also have water as their dispersion medium and are available in either sheets or gels (e.g. Scherisorb*, Intrasite gel*, Gelliperm and Vigilon).
- Polysaccharides or xerogels are sterile, spherical beads of dextranomer which absorb wound exudate (e.g. Debrisan* and Idosorb*).
- Foam dressings are used as cavity fillers due to their absorbency (e.g. lyofoam* and allevyn).
- Semi-permeable films are made from polyurethane and are water-tight dressings which act as a barrier over the wound (e.g. Tegaderm*, Opsite and Bioclusive).
- Low-Adherent dressings (e.g. Melolin* and NA*) are suitable for use on dry wounds or as secondary dressings.

Only a small sample of the numerous wound care products available are mentioned here, a full list with descriptions can be found in Morgans, *Formulary of wound management products* (1992a). Up-to-date information regarding availability on Drug Tariff can be obtained through reference to the *General Practitioners' Drug Tariff Handbook*.

Treatment of infected wounds

Before a diagnosis of wound infection is made, a combination of clinical signs should be observed, rather than relying solely on the evidence produced by a wound swab. The early detection of wound infection is important, not only because it prolongs the inflammatory stage of wound healing, but also because it is likely to cause discomfort for the patient.

There does not appear to be a place for the use of topical antibiotics in wound care as they carry the risk of resistance, emergence of new organisms and allergy. An invasive infection requires treatment in order for healing to take place. Systemic antibiotics are recommended for patients with definite clinical signs of infection (Leaper, 1992).

Pain relief

The importance of adequate pain control for patients with chronic wounds should not be underestimated, as pain may lead to long-term demoralisation and depression. Judkins (1992) suggests that analgesia should be administered regularly rather than on an as-required basis, and suggests non-steriodal anti-inflammatory drugs like Ibobruffen may be suitable. Anxiety needs support and information-giving. Anti-depressant drugs may also have a place in the management of chronic wound pain. Finally the choice of dressing may influence wound pain. Traditional dressings have been found to be more painful when in situ, as well as at dressing changes, than the modern dressings such as semi-permeable films, alginates and hydrocolloids, although the reasons for this is not clearly understood. The choice of dressing may therefore not only influence healing, but reduce the need for analgesia.

(*Indicates availability on Drug Tariff and therefore prescribable by patients' GPs, The list of products available is regularily updated).

The control of odour is not only a consideration for wound healing but is also an important consideration for the maintainance of the dignity and well-being of the patient.

Treatment of venous leg ulcers

The aim in the management of venous leg ulcers is to increase deep venous return and reduce the venous hypertension. In addition to local wound management, this can be achieved in the ambulant resident by compression therapy together with periods of leg elevation (Cameron, 1994). A correctly applied compression bandage will support the superficial veins and help prevent capillary leakage, reduce tissue oedema and improve the tone of the calf muscle. Compression bandages should be applied when the limb is least oedematous, with the patient sitting down. The leg should be supported in an extended position with the foot at right angles to the limb.

The bandage should be applied from the base of the toes to the tibial tuberositity just below the knee, using a spiral technique. Studies have shown that compression applied in a decreasing gradient up the leg will produce an increase in the blood flow velocity. The bandage should be applied maintaining an even extension and a 50 per cent overlap. This is a skilled procedure which will require staff training. Since most venous ulcers are treated in the community the community nursing service may provide a useful resource. The ideal pressure for healing to take place is generally considered to be between 25–40 mm Hg at the ankle, reducing over the calf.

Bandages have been subdivided into four categories based on their ability to retain predetermined levels of tension under controlled laboratory conditions. They are light compression (14–17 mmHg at the ankle), moderate compression (18–24 mm Hg at the ankle), high compression (25–35 mm Hg at the ankle) and extra high compression (60 mmHg at the ankle). A variety of these bandages are available on the Drug Tariff. Details of comparative evaluations of different bandages available are reviewed by Cullum (1994).

A check should be undertaken again 24 hours after the application of the compression bandage. After the initial reduction in tissue oedema, bandage changes may be extended up to one week. If, after a period of 4–6 weeks, healing is not progressing it is imperative that a review must take place.

Many different bandaging regimes are used and are basically fall into three categories, elastic or short-stretch compression bandages; support bandaging regimes consisting of paste bandages and outer support bandages to improve calf muscle function; and support stockings or preshaped tubular bandages. The importance of assessment (already described) prior to treatment is stressed as, if compression is applied to a limb that has an impaired arterial blood supply, it would compromise the blood supply and have the potential to cause serious damage (Cherry, Cameron and Ryan, 1991).

The pharmacological agent oxpentifylline, has been shown to have a beneficial role in treating ulcers by improving the delivery of oxygen to ischaemic tissues (James, Holland, Hughes et al., 1984). A more recent controlled study showed that oxpentifylline also improved healing in venous leg ulcers (Colgan, Dormandy, Jones et al.,1990).

All wound dressings should be used in accordance with the manufacturer's instructions and changed as infrequently as possible. The regimes will need to be reviewed in accordance with the stage of healing. If improvement is not achieved after a reasonable interval or if it is not sustained, treatment needs to be reviewed and a more suitable regime implemented. In the case of chronic non-healing wounds the advice of a wound care specialist or vascular or dermatological specialist may be appropriate. This should be arranged following consultation with the patient's GP.

Access to the latest and best treatments may be obtainable for patients with serious wound healing problems by their referral to a specialist wound healing clinic, for example that described by Miller (1994a) at a tissue repair research unit.

The long-term existence of chronic wounds cannot be justified without all possible sources of help having been sought. As already discussed, the registered nurse is accountable not only for her practice but for her omissions (UKCC, 1992a), and is therefore responsible for eliciting whatever assistance may be necessary in order for treatment goals to be achieved.

Guidelines for future practice

The NHS Executive drew up clinical guidelines on the prevention and management of pressure sores in March, 1994, and, following their testing in three pilot sites, they are due to be released shortly. They are the result of the consensus of a multi-disciplinary panel of experts and cover areas such as classification of pressure sores, risk assessment and audit. It is intended that the guidelines will suggest to nurses what comprises good care and how to provide it.

It is suggested that every unit implements a strategy for the prevention and management of wounds. The objectives are to work as a disiplinary team in order to raise awareness by assessing and addressing areas of concern, to standardise methods of treatment and care based on available resources and research findings and to provide written guidelines and protocols for pressure sore prevention and wound management. The latter may either be formulated locally or the existing policy of a health authority or trust adopted. A guide as to how to develop a wound care policy is available (Morgan, 1992b).

Conclusions

Nurses working in care homes aim to provide the best possible quality of life for their patients. If this is to be achieved patient care must be of a high standard, which includes pressure sore prevention and the treatment of wounds. In order for this to be acheived, nurses not only need to have up-to-date knowledge and a high level of skill, but also the equipment necessary. They are likely to be required to advise GPs on the prescription of the most appropriate treatments and nursing home owners on investment in pressure-relieving devices.

Useful contacts

The Tissue Viability Society, c/o Wessex Rehabilitation Association, Odstock Hospital, Salisbury SP2 8BJ.
The Wound Care Society, PO Box 263, Northampton NN3 4UJ.

Journals

Journal of Tissue Viability. Tissue Viability Society.
Wound Management. Media Medica.
Journal of Wound Care. Macmillan Magazines.
Nursing Journal of the Tissue Viability Society. Supplement in Nursing Standard.

References

Altmeyer, P. (1993) Research results being ignored. *Nursing Standard*, **7**, 21, 13.
Ayton, M. (1985) Wounds that won't heal. *Nursing Times*, **81**, 46, 16-19.
Bethell, E. (1994) The development of a strategy for the prevention and management of pressure sores. *Journal of Wound Care*, **3**, 7, 342–343.
Boardman, M., Melhuish, J.M. and Harding, K.G. (1994) Hue, saturation and intensity in the healing wound image. *Journal of Wound Care*, **3**, 7, 314–319.
Bloomsbury and Islington Health Authority, Directorate of Community Health Services (1991) Community Nurse Wound Management Policy.
Brennan, S.S., Foster, M.E., and Leaper, D.J. (1986) Antiseptics toxicity in wound healing by secondary intention. *Journal of Hospital Infection*, **8**, 3, 263–267.
Brennan, S.S. and Leaper, D.J. (1985) The effect of antiseptics on the healing wound: a study using rabbit earchamber. *British Journal of Surgery*, **72**, 10, 780–782.
Bridel, J. (1992) Pressure sore development and intra-operative risk. *Nursing Standard*, **7**, 5, 28–30.
Bridel, J. (1993) The epidemiology of pressure sores. *Nursing Standard*, **7**, 42, 25–30.
Callam, M.J. (1992) Prevalence of Chronic Leg Ulceration and Severe Chronic Venous Disease in Western Countries. *Phlebology Supplement*, **1**, 6–12.

Callam, M.J., Harper, D.R, Dale, J.J. and Ruckley, C.V. (1987a) Arterial disease in chronic leg ulceration: an underestimated hazard? Lothian and Forth Valley leg ulcer study. *British Medical Journal of Clinical Research.*, **294**, (6577), 929–931.

Callam, M.J., Harper, D.R. and Dale, J.J. (1987b) Chronic ulcer of the leg: clinical history. *British Medical Journal of Clinical Research*, **294**, (6584), 1389–91.

Cameron, J. (1994). Venous leg ulcers. *Elderly Care*, **6**, 5, 23–26.

Cherry, G.W., Cameron, J. and Ryan, T.J. (1991) *Leg Ulcer Blueprint. Treatment and the prevention of recurrence.* Uxbridge: Convatec.

Cherry, G.W. and Ryan, T.J. (1985). Enhanced wound angiogenesis with a new hydrocolloid dressing. In: T.J. Ryan (ed.) *An environment for healing: the role of occlusion.* (International Congress and Symposium Series. No 88). London: Royal Society of Medicine.

Clark, M. (1994). Top nurse calls for a halt to pressure sore research. *Nursing Standard*, **8**, 40, 14.

Colgan, M.P., Dormandy, J.A., Jones, P.W. et al. (1990) Oxpentifylline treatment of venous ulcers of the leg. *British Medical Journal*, **300**, 972–975.

Collier, M. (1994). Assessing a wound. RCN Nursing Update. *Nursing Standard*, **8**, 49, 3–8.

Cullum, N. (1994). The nursing management of leg ulcers in the community: A critical review of the research. Department of Nursing, University of Liverpool.

Department of Health (1991) *The Health of the Nation: a strategy for health in England.* London: HMSO.

Department of Health (1993). Pressure Sores – A Key Quality Indicator. London: HMSO.

Flannigan, M. (1990) Wound Assessment Educational Leaflet, 4. Wound Care Society.

Flannigan, M. (1994) Assessment driteria. *Nursing Times*, **90**, 35, 76–88.

Fletcher, J. (1994) Pressure sore prevention. *Nursing Times*, **90**, 24, 76.

Gawkrodger, D.J, (1992) *Skin ageing and itching in the elderly.* Nursing Dialogue. No 11. Barrie Rowen Associates.

Heng, M.C.Y., Pilgrim, J.P., and Beck, F.W.J.A. (1984). A simplified hyperbaric oxygen technique for leg ulcers. *Archives of Dermatology*, **120**, 640–645.

James, D, Holland, B., Hughes, M. et al. (1984) Oxpentifylline: effects on red cell deformability and oxygen availability from blood in intermittent claudication. *Clinical Haemorrheology*, **4**, 525–531.

Johnson, A. (1988) The cleansing ethic. *Nursing Times. Community Outlook Supplement*, **84**, 6, 9–10.

Judkins, K. (1992) Analgesia and analgesics in wound management. In Proceedings, Going into the 90's: The Pharmacist and Woundcare. Eurosciences Communication.

King's Fund Centre (1989) *The prevention and management of pressure sores within Health Districts.* London: King's Fund Centre.

Lawerence, J.C., Lilly, H.A. and Kidson, A. (1994) A novel presentation of saline for wound irrigation. *Journal of Wound Care*, **3**, 7, 334–337.

Layton, A.M., Ibbotson, S.H., Davies, J.A. et al. (1994) Randomised trial of oral aspirin for chronic venous leg ulcers. *The Lancet*, **344**, 8916, 164–165.

Leaper, D. (1992). The use of antiseptics and antibiotics in wound care. In: Proceedings, Going into the 90s: The Pharmacist and Woundcare. Eurosciences Communication.

Leaper, D.J. and Simpson, R.A. (1986) The effect of antiseptics and topical antimicrobals on wound healing. *Journal of Antimicrobial Chemotherapy*, **17**, 2, 131–137.

Lester, R. (1992) The aetiology of pressure sores. In Proceedings, Going into the 90's: The pharmacist and Wound Care. Eurosciences Communication.

Lewis, C. (1994) Bound to heal. *The Monitor*, Winter, p. 6.

Melzack, R. (1975). The McGill Pain Questionaire. *Pain*, **1**, 3, 277–299.

Miller, M. (1994a) Setting up a nurse-led clinic in wound healing. *Nursing Standard*, **9**, 6, 54–56.

Miller, M. (1994b) The ideal healing environment. *Nursing Times*, **90**, 45, 62–68.

Moffatt, C. (1994) The hazards of poor assessment. *Nursing Standard*, **9**, 6, 53.

Moody, M., Fanale, J.E., Thompson, M. *et al* (1988) Impact of staff education on pressure sore development in elderly hospitalised patients. *Archives of Internal Medicine*, **148**, 10, 2241–2243.

Moody, M. (1992) The evolving role of the nurse. *Wound Management*, **2**, 4, 3.

Moody, M. (1993) State of the art of wound care. A survey of wound management practice in nursing homes. Wound care in the community. *Professional Nurse Supplement*, p. 7–11.

Morgan, D.A. (1992a) *Formulary of wound management products. A guide for health care staff* (5th edition). Media Medica Publications.

Morgan, D.A.(1992b) *A wound management formulary. A guide on how to develop a wound care policy*. Convatec.

Morison, M.J. (1990a) *Pressure Sore Blue Print: Aetiology, Prevention and Management*. Convatec Ltd.

Morison, M.J. (1990b) Wound cleansing – which solution? *Nursing Standard*, **4**, 52.

Morison, M.J. (1994) Wound Care: A problem solving approach. RCN Nursing Update. *Nursing Standard*, **8**, 19, 3–8.

Murray, Y. (1988) Tradition rather than cure? *Nursing Times*, **84**, 38, 75–80.

Norton, D. (1962) An investigation of geriatric nursing problems in hospital. National Corporation for the Care of Old People. Hong Kong.

Pudner, R. (1994) Wound care in three European Countries. *Nursing Standard*, **8**, 48, 50–51.

Robert, R. (1994) Pressure sore care in Clyd nursing homes. *Journal of Wound Care*, **3**, 8, 385–387.

Reid, J. and Morison, M. (1994) Classification of pressure sore severity. *Nursing Times*, **90**, 20, 46–49.

Roper, N., Logan, W., and Tierney, A, (1980) The Elements of Nursing. Edinburgh: Churchill Livingstone.

Royal Marsden Hospital (1990). Dont's. ENB 285.

Stotts, N.A. (1988) Predicting Pressure Ulcer Development in Surgical Patients. *Heart and Lung*, **17**, 641–647.

Touche Ross (1993) *The Costs of Pressure Sores*. London: Touche Ross.

Tsukada, K, Tokunaja, K. and Iwana, T. et al. (1992) The pH changes of pressure ulcers related to the healing process of wounds. *Wounds: A Compendium of Clinical Research and Practice*, **4**, 1, 16–20.

Turner, T., Schmidt, R. and Harding, K. (1986) *Advances in wound management. Symposium Proceedings, Cardiff*. John Wiley and Sons.

UKCC (1992a) Code of Professional Conduct. London: United Kingdom Central Council for Nursing, Midwifery and Health Visiting.

UKCC (1992b) Scope of Professional Practise: A Position Statement. London: United Kingdom Central Council for Nursing, Midwifery and Health Visiting.

University of Dundee (1993) *The Wound Handbook*. Centre for Medical Education, Dundee, in conjunction with Perspective, London.

Varghese, M.C,. Arthur, K.B., Canter, M. and Callweed, D. (1986). Local environment of chronic wounds under synthetic dressings. *Archives of Dermatology*, **122**, 52–57.

Wagner, F.W. (1981) The dysvascular foot: a system for diagnosis and treatment. *Foot Ankle*, **2**, 64.

Waterlow, J. (1988) The Waterlow card for the prevention and management of pressure sores: towards a pocket policy. *CARE – Science and Practice*, **6**(1), 8–12.

Wilson, E. (1989) Prevention and treatment of leg ulcers. *Health Trends*, **21**, 97.

Young, J. (1990) News from the society (Tissue Viability Society). *Nursing Standard*, **8**, 48, 45.

Young, M. (1993) *Diabetic foot ulceration blueprint. A guide for the primary health care team*. Convatec.

16

Supportive Activities and Symptom Relief

Glenda Hunter and Hazel Heath

Introduction

Health and well-being normally vary constantly throughout life, and each individual places his or her personal values on health, or particular aspects of health. In terms of maintaining a constancy of health and well-being, the changes which accompany ageing offer challenges to all of us, and we tend to experience some limitations in performance as we grow older. Some changes in physical capacity associated with muscle strength, pulmonary function, cardiac output or kidney efficiency, may not seriously interfere with a person's ability to function in day-to-day life, but they can disrupt the body's steady physiological balance, and make it more difficult for the body to maintain its homeostasis (equilibrium).

In older age, the multiple and complex changes of ageing can mean that ill-health presents differently (altered presentation of disease), and that diseases are multiple (multiple pathology). In addition, health status interacts with the social changes which accompany ageing, and the psychological adjustment to these.

Older people living in care homes tend to have some of the most complex and multiple health care needs of any group in society. Many of them will experience major illnesses, others chronic ill-health or disability. In addition, they may experience age-related changes which interfere with daily living.

This chapter reviews some common physiological age-related symptoms which may trouble older people who live in care homes, and offers ideas for symptom relief and supportive activities. It considers some complementary, supplementary or alternative therapies that nurses in care homes can use to help relieve unpleasant symptoms and enhance the well-being of the older people with whom they work. Lastly it highlights particular considerations concerning medications and older people, and reviews the role of the care home nurse in ordering, storing and administering drugs.

Common symptoms in older people

Some of the common symptoms experienced by older people are discussed in other chapters. These include difficulty walking (Chapter 13:

Mobility), depression, mental confusion (see Chapter 11: Mental Health), sight and hearing problems (see Chapter 10: Communication, and Chapter 7: Home Life), cognitive changes (see Chapter 9: Educational Issues), difficulties associated with eating (see Chapter 12: Nutrition), continence problems and constipation (see Chapter 14: Continence).

Others include shortness of breath, pain, and sexual difficulties.

Shortness of breath

Shortness of breath may be one of the first indicators of ageing changes, particularly when an older person is faced with unusual or stressful situations which increase the body's demand for oxygen.

An older person's respiratory health will to some extent have been determined by his or her lifestyle in terms of occupation, exposure to environmental pollutants, and smoking habits. Many older people have at some time in their lives smoked cigarettes, or been exposed to pulmonary irritants, such as asbestos or coal.

Due to lung tissue changes, and also decreased cardiac output, the efficiency of the lungs, and the uptake of oxygen, are reduced in older people. Diminished immune system response, and a less efficient self-cleansing action of the respiratory cilia, contribute to a lowered resistance to infection. Common problems experienced by older people include a reduced capacity for physical exertion, shortness of breath, dizziness, coughing, wheezing, or recurrent chest infections.

Nurses can help relieve symptoms by encouraging the older person to maintain an upright posture, setting the shoulder girdle to allow maximum capacity with minimum effort, deep (diaphragmatic) breathing, avoiding pulmonary irritants (such as cigarette smoke or dust), maintaining adequate fluid intake, exercising to maximum capacity, influenza vaccinations, and seeking medical advice for respiratory tract infections.

Pain

The physical discomforts, aches or pains experienced in older age can severely limit day-to-day activities, and the enjoyment of life. Pain can arise as a consequence of many factors, including psychological stressors or anxiety, and the experience of pain is complicated by age-related changes (particularly in the nervous system), generational beliefs, and cultural influences.

Pain may manifest differently in older adults. For example, chest pain may be a sign of arthritis of the spine, herpes zoster infection or an abdominal disorder. However, the characteristic chest pain experienced by younger adults with myocardial infarction, may be absent in older people, giving rise to the 'silent MI' (White, 1995).

Older people may not report pain because they believe it to be an inevitable part of ageing, or because they fear illness, loss of independence, or death (Herr and Mobily, 1991). Alternatively, McCaffery and Beebe (1994) suggest that older people may believe that it is not acceptable to show pain, and may use a variety of mechanisms to distract attention from their discomfort.

The emotional component of the pain experience in older age may also be distinct. Schultz (1982) suggests that older people in pain simultaneously experience many different emotions which are linked to their accumulation of life experiences.

Pain in older people may not only result in physical incapacity, but also poor self-image, low self-esteem or depression. It is important therefore for nurses to be vigilant for pain, to take any complaints of pain seriously, and to consider the older person's psychological and emotional needs as well as the relief of their physical pain.

An individual's experience of pain can be affected by anxiety, fatigue, previous experiences, coping style, degree of perceived control, degree of attention to pain, and available support.

Pain-relieving measures include:

- a review, with the person of the causes of their pain, e.g. muscle spasm. This understanding can help the individual to avoid pain-inducing anxiety;
- emotional support;
- avoiding additional problems by maintaining the body's normal functioning (e.g. promoting sleep and avoiding constipation);
- positioning painful limbs so that they are supported and comfortable;
- warm baths;
- hot or cold pads;
- the application of liniment;
- touch;
- massage and aromatherapy;
- acupressure or acupuncture;
- reflexology;
- distraction;
- relaxation and guided imagery;
- anticipatory guidance (helping the older person to anticipate a pain experience in order to reduce anxiety and cognitively gain a level of pain relief) (Walding, 1991);
- biofeedback (a behavioural therapy in which information is given to the individual about his/her physical responses (e.g. blood pressure) and ways to exercise voluntary control over those responses);
- TENS (transcutaneous electrical nerve stimulation), which stimulates the nerves beneath the skin with a mild electrical current from electrodes placed near to the pain site. In Taylor et al's. (1983) study, people who received TENS reported greater pain relief than people who received opioid analgesics. Physiologically, TENS works effectively with older people, but, because the skin of older people is more fragile, they may experience skin problems, depending on where the electrodes are placed;
- pharmacological management with analgesics (e.g. paracetamol), co-analgesics (e.g. diazepam), anti-inflammatory agents (e.g. indometacin), opiods (e.g. dihydrocodeine or diamorphine hydrochloride). Patient-controlled analgesia (PCA) can be given via a pump.

Sexual difficulties

Sexual activity in later life can be affected by debilitating, immobilising or painful illnesses, but it can also be affected by pharmacological treatments, particularly for such conditions as hypertension and angina, or by the inconsiderate use of catheters or other appliances (Riley, 1994, Kellett, 1989).

In men, normal age-related changes may result in a prolonged time to achieve erection, a reduced ejaculatory frequency, and a longer recovery period. In women, vaginal dryness or atrophy can be problematic. However, for older people living in care homes, the major barriers to sexual expression may be the narrow, negative or stereotypical staff attitudes which can severely restrict, or even totally curtail, this aspect of older people's lives. Falk and Falk's (1980) study concluded that the prevention of sexual expression in care homes is achieved in three ways:

● It is condemned by societal and staff attitudes.
● It is prevented by restrictive care home regimes.
● The assumptions that sex is inappropriate or 'dirty' for older people are internalised by the residents themselves.

Despite physical frailty, many older people would want to continue to be sexually active. In White's (1982) 250 interviews of nursing home residents in Texas, 17 per cent said they would like to be sexually active if they could find a partner or suitable accommodation, and 9 per cent were sexually active. The average age of the interviewees was 82.

In order to be supportive of older people's choices, nurses in care homes should:

● examine their own attitudes to sexual, and sexuality expression in older age;
● examine their own attitudes to heterosexuality, homosexuality and bisexuality;
● review the facilities they offer in the home, and particularly for privacy; for example glass panels in doors which allow staff to see whatever is happening within a resident's room (Counsel and Care, 1991);
● review care regimes which allow no time for residents to be alone (for example to masturbate) or to spend uninterrupted time with partners;
● learn about the normal age-related changes in sexual response, in order that they can sensitively broach this subject with residents at appropriate opportunities;
● review medications which may reduce physiological arousal (such as analgesics or antidepressants), increase arousal (such as levodopa), or cause erectile impotence (such as anticholinergics, beta blockers or diuretics). Other medications causing problems include anti-hypertensives, sedatives and tranquillisers, sexual hormone preparations (such as stilboestrol), anticonvulsants, and alcohol;
● if there are problems, check whether the person has undergone surgery such as prostatectomy, any radical pelvic surgery, aortoiliac surgery, or sympathectomy;

- try to avoid using catheters if people are sexually active, or teach them how to manage the catheter during sexual intercourse;
- avoid using incontinence pads which might impair sexual activity; and
- try to be open-minded and non-judgemental.

As Comfort states (1982) 'Old persons in institutions should enjoy, so far as is possible, the same freedom of sexual choice which adults enjoy in society at large, and should not be considered senile, or sedated, in response to the sexual attitudes of staff'.

Supportive activities

Nurses in care homes have used many creative and innovative means of maintaining the health and well-being of their residents, and minimising unpleasant symptoms. A pleasant, meaningful and active environment, both physically and psychosocially (see Chapter 7: Home Life), and the facilitation of individual rights and choices (see Chapter 6: Rights, Risks and Responsibilities) can help older people maintain a positive sense of control and meaning in life. Helping to maintain a balance in life between managing ill-health and encouraging the older person's contribution to life, between rest and activity, between solitude and company, and between seriousness and laughter, can also help to minimise problems.

Laughter serves as a psychological and physical release. Research has demonstrated that, in older people, laughter stimulates the production of hormones that enhance feelings of well-being, improve pain tolerance, reduce anxiety, facilitate respiratory relaxation and enhance metabolism (Sullivan and Deane 1988, Williams 1986). Sullivan and Deane also found that, as a result of humour, older people tend to be more self-disclosing and willing to share concerns of deeper significance. This can help to enhance the nurses' effectiveness in providing emotional support to older people, and to humanise the experience of illness (Dugan, 1989).

Complementary, supplementary and supportive therapies

Complementary therapies are increasingly being used in care homes, where they can be of tremendous benefit to the residents and the staff. Nurses are increasingly becoming interested in complementary therapies, and many have taken additional training (Rankin-Box, 1992).

Complementary therapies are distinct from conventional medicine, which uses a dynamic interventionist approach to alleviate suffering by controlling symptoms of disease processes diagnosed through pathology. Complementary, alternative or supplementary therapies view symptoms as having accumulated over time and through mismanagement of health-related behaviour or lifestyle. These therapies therefore aim to recruit the self-healing capacities of the body by amplifying the natural recuperative processes and by augmenting the energies upon which the individual's health depends (Cooke, 1995). They relate 'directly to an adaptation process to promote a harmony with that person's surroundings' (Fulder, 1989).

Despite many strong advocates for complementary therapies, they have not received universal acceptance, particularly from the medical profession. There are two major difficulties with this. The first is that robust research into the health gain outcomes, or effects, of complementary therapies is still developing. The second is that the regulation of complementary practices is incomplete, although the Institute of Complementary Medicine has now established a Register of Complementary Practitioners in order to define training criteria which conform to EC directives, and to establish criteria for membership of the British register.

There are many different courses offering training and education for various complementary therapies, and some are described in the Institute of Complementary Medicine publications. In January 1993, the European Community declared that training courses for all therapies should be of at least three years in length. Some colleges provide three year courses with degree status, and many colleges of nursing provide courses with university accreditation. These courses do not necessarily train nurses to practice the therapies but do enable them to respond to the patient's questions and needs and to evaluate the effectiveness and appropriateness of various therapies (Trevelyan and Booth, 1994). There are also plans for NVQ competency standards for complementary therapists.

In its 'principles on the use of complementary therapies', the UKCC (1994) stated that 'complementary therapies are increasingly finding a more substantial role within health care. It is vital that nurses ensure that the introduction of these therapies as adjuncts to the range of nursing care is always made in the best interests of patients and clients'. The statement referred to the Code (1992a) and Scope of Professional Conduct (1992b, paragraphs 8–11), and the Standards for the Administration of Medicines (UKCC, 1992c, paragraphs 37 and 38). The UKCC position is that it is the responsibility of the individual practitioner to judge whether a qualification obtained in complementary therapy has brought him or her to an appropriate level of competence to use the skill in patient or client care. The UKCC reinforces that the nurse must honestly acknowledge any limits of personal knowledge, skill and competence in all areas of practice, decline any duties or responsibilities unless able to perform them in a safe and skilled manner, and take steps to remedy any deficits in knowledge and skills. The registered nurse is personally accountable for all aspects of his or her practice (see Chapter 3: Professional Nursing Issues). It is also an important to professional teamwork to discuss the use of complementary therapies with the doctor and any other colleagues in the health care team for a particular person. The UKCC suggests that employers may wish to develop local policies to provide frameworks for the use of complementary therapies.

The Royal College of Nursing has issued guidelines to assist nurses in selecting complementary therapy courses, and the RCN indemnity insurance scheme covers the majority of these, except herbalism and homeopathy. The RCN Complementary Therapies in Nursing Membership

Group organises conferences, and issues newsletters to keep its members up to date on UK activities.

Nurses are not able to advertise as nurses if they are using their therapeutic skills as part of their practice repertoire. In 1993, the International Council for Nursing proposed that nurses should be allowed to practice their profession outside the NHS as independent practitioners, but this issue is as yet unresolved (Cooke 1995).

Complementary therapies in care homes

A variety of therapies are currently in use in care homes around the country, and a selection are described below. When considering the use of such therapies, however, it is important to recognise that people from some cultural or religious groups may find their use offensive. For example, if individuals believe that the life force emanates from a deity, they may object to a therapy which focuses on a life force within human beings.

Useful therapies for care homes include relaxation, distraction, guided imagery, touch, massage, aromatherapy, acupressure and reflexology.

Relaxation, distraction and guided imagery

Relaxation is an active process which aims to put the body into a resting state. Various techniques can be used, including music, talking tapes, meditation, yoga and progressive muscle relaxation exercises. Relaxation can help to relieve tension and pain. It can be practised indefinitely and seems to have no side effects.

During a relaxed state, distraction can be used to focus the attention of the individual on a pleasurable stimulus or activity such as a picture, music, singing or praying. Distraction can help enhance relaxation and relieve pain, and is effective for short periods.

In guided imagery, the person focuses on a pleasurable or helpful mental image, which is progressed under the guidance of the nurse or therapist. For example, each intake of breath could be imaged as dissolving pain or tension in a particular part of the body.

It is important that the images and distractions used are derived from the person's individual, cultural and religious beliefs.

Therapeutic touch

There are many different types of touch, and each can convey a different message (see Chapter 10: Communication). Therapeutic touch is an ancient therapy based on the philosophy that living beings are energy fields that interact with a universal life force in the environment. Ill-health results from problems with energy flow, and the therapist draws energy from the environment and from areas of the client's body where there is congestion, to direct them towards areas lacking in energy. When the energy balance is restored, the body can regenerate its wholeness, and regain its vital energy.

It is not necessary to have skin-to-skin contact in therapeutic touch, as the energy field radiates beyond the skin surface (Sayre-Adams, 1993). It can therefore be particularly beneficial to older people who are unable to maintain a specific bodily positioning for any length of time. Therapeutic touch has been beneficial in the relief of stress and tension headaches (Sayre-Adams, 1994) and in mental health settings (Hill and Oliver, 1993).

Therapeutic massage

This is a technique that uses a variety of manual movements, and degrees of pressure. In moving the soft tissues and muscles in particular areas of the body, it is claimed that the circulation of blood and lymph is stimulated, and that toxins are cleared.

Massage can aid relaxation and may be used to treat people with hypertension, constipation, depression, tension, anxiety, insomnia, headaches and asthma. It can also be effective in enhancing self-esteem and self-confidence (Sanderson and Carter, 1994).

Massage can enhance the therapeutic relationship with patients/clients (Sanderson and Carter, 1994) but, because the process may release emotions, it is important that the environment and time allowed for the therapy be appropriate.

Some general precautions are necessary when undertaking massage. For example:

- Special care must be taken to avoid contact with skin surface problems, e.g. varicose veins, scar tissue, bruising or tender inflamed areas, (a very light touch may be used (e.g. petrissage), or just holding the hands away from the area of skin and maintaining the massage movements).
- People receiving anticoagulation therapy at high risk of subcutaneous haemorrhage should not be given massage.
- Skin lesions, and a site of a recent fracture should be avoided.
- Massage may speed the effects of drugs.

In addition, there are some special considerations for older people:

- The position for massage may need to be adapted, for example, for people who have had strokes, who are in wheelchairs, or who are unable to lie comfortably for any length of time.
- The skin of older people may be more friable, and likely to be damaged if not treated gently, for example from jewellery.

Massage therapy was introduced in our nursing home approximately three years ago. We found that residents responded to touch and the massaging of creams into their skin to alleviate dryness. Four nurses have now been trained in massage therapy and we have devised a standard on massage therapy for frail older people.

We have found that, as well as being relaxing, massage has a calming effect on our residents. They say that it helps them with sleeping problems, and helps to relieve discomfort in damaged limbs. We have also found it effective in calming one resident who has a tendency to become agitated and disruptive. Massaging hands which were contracted from muscle wastage and nerve damage following strokes has also been particularly effective in that residents have not only gained relief from discomfort, but have found themselves more able to use the hand.

Aromatherapy

'Aromatherapy is an ancient healing practice ... which uses essential oils extracted from plants to provide psychological and physiological healing' (Cooke, 1995). The oil is believed to represent the life-force of the plant, tree or shrub, and each has its distinct personality, odour and healing properties. Some oils may stimulate, others sedate. The oils may be used in massage, or to permeate the atmosphere.

Most people find essential oils relaxing but they should be used with caution. Some aromas can cause nausea, or may evoke bad memories rather than pleasant ones. Aromatic oils may not be appropriate for use in conjunction with chemotherapy or other treatments and, because it is difficult to control the drift of an aroma, they should be used with caution in public places, and only with sufficient ventilation. Essential oils should never be used neat, with the exception of lavender, and many aromatherapists recommend that they should not be taken internally. Oils should not be used directly on bruised or broken skin, unless specifically recommended (e.g. lavender).

In addition to the massage precautions for older people, it should be remembered that because of age-related changes, older people may react to some oils in the same way as they react to drugs. Strong oils and multiple mixtures of oils should not be used on frail older people.

For the clients in our home, grapeseed and lavender are the most commonly used. Lavender is very versatile and has seemed to be suitable for almost everyone. It has been particularly effective to relieve headaches, even migraines, and for insomnia and to heal skin from, for example, burns.

Reflexology

The principles are based on the belief from Ancient Chinese philosophy that the body's natural healing can be enhanced by applying pressure to certain areas of the feet and hands. These areas are said to be connected by a flow of energy through channels or meridians. The therapist identifies crystalline deposits in certain areas of the foot (which relate to an organ of the body) that are impeding the flow of energy. Treatment consists of gently dispersing these deposits with firm massage of the identified area of the foot.

Reflexology is believed to be beneficial for gastrointestinal disorders (such as heartburn, constipation and diarrhoea), skin problems such as eczema or psoriasis) arthritis, asthma and migraines (Trevelyan and Booth, 1994).

Although reflexology is considered to be a safe procedure, contra-indications include deep vein thrombosis, leg ulcers, pronounced varicose veins, viral infections, fungal disease (such as athlete's foot) phlebitis or other circulatory disorder of the lower limbs. It should be used with caution in people who have gallstones, kidney stones, liver problems or a pacemaker.

Acupressure

As with reflexology and acupuncture, acupressure aims to work on the energy flows within the meridians of the body. It works on the same basis as acupuncture but without the needles. Pressure is applied with the fingers for 3–5 seconds at specific points along the meridians. This aims to remove energy blockages and open the meridians so that energy can flow unhindered, thus promoting good health.

Acupressure is thought to be particularly effective for constipation, headaches, insomnia, sciatica, gastrointestinal disorders, arthritis, back pain and muscle cramps. The treatment has few reported adverse effects, but should be used with caution with people who have acute illness. Pressures will also need to be adjusted for older people who are physically frail or disabled.

Pharmacological symptom relief

Medications can be extremely effective in controlling and relieving symptoms but special considerations are necessary when administering drugs to older people, and nurses in care homes carry the prime responsibility for identifying and dealing with any problems which may arise.

Drug therapy and older people

Older people are particularly at risk from drugs-related problems. There are several reasons for this:

● Complex disease patterns in older age can make diagnosis difficult.
● Multiple pathology can result in multiple prescriptions (polypharmacy).
● Polypharmacy can result in adverse interactions between the various drugs.
● Negative attitudes to older people can result in unnecessary and inappropriate prescriptions.
● Older people are thus prescribed more drugs than younger people.
● The incidence of non-compliance is high in older people, for various reasons.

In addition, age-related changes affect the way drugs are processed through the body. Pharmacokinetics is the study of how drugs enter the body, reach their site of action, are metabolised, and exit the body (Webster, 1995).

Age-related changes affect drug absorption, distribution, metabolism and excretion.

Absorption: This is the passage of the drug into the bloodstream. Changes in the gastrointestinal tract can affect the degree and rate of absorption. The loss of elasticity in oral mucosa, delayed oesophageal clearance due to weakened contractions, decreased gastric acidity and peristalsis in older people can result in difficulty swallowing drugs, sensitivity, irritation or tissue erosion in the mouth or oesophagus, and altered solubility of certain drugs.

The absorption of injected drugs can be affected by reduced muscle mass and reduced blood circulation (exacerbated by muscle inactivity).

For locally or topically administered drugs, reduced skin cell turnover, moisture and elasticity can result in local irritation, damage or bleeding. The result is delayed and unpredictable absorption of a drug, and it is appropriate to give smaller doses in most cases.

Distribution: A drug's distribution is affected by the physiological make-up of the individual and the properties of the drug. Most medications are distributed to body fat or water. The less a person weighs, the greater the concentration of the drug in the tissues, and the effects of the drug are more powerful. Older adults experience changes in fat:protein:tissue ratio, with proportionately less water, more fat, and often a reduction in height. Some drugs bind to skeletal muscle, and one of these is digoxin. If a person loses skeletal muscle, this can increase the availability of digoxin.

The concentration of a drug at a specific site depends on the number of blood vessels in the tissues. Vascular efficiency may be reduced in older age. A reduced cardiac output may also affect drug distribution.

Most medications bind to some extent with the proteins, particularly albumin, in the blood. When bound, they are not pharmacologically active. However, older people have decreased levels of albumin, and 'free' amounts of a drug are therefore increased. Because of this, older people may be particularly at risk of an increase in drug activity, toxicity, or both (Webster, 1995).

Metabolism: This is a process which, after the drug reaches its site of action, converts it into an inactive form which can be excreted easily. Most of this process takes place in the liver, where the enzymes detoxify, degrade, and remove biologically active chemicals. With age, the reduced blood flow and enzyme production in the liver result in a slowing of the metabolism, which causes drugs to accumulate in the body.

Elimination: Small amounts of drug may be excreted through saliva and perspiration, but the main route for excretion is via the kidneys or the gastrointestinal tract. Kidney filtration decreases with ageing, and drugs may accumulate in the body, causing toxicity. Maintaining an adequate fluid intake can assist drug elimination, but it may be necessary to reduce the dose. Older people on long-term or multiple drug therapy are therefore particularly at risk.

Precautions when administering drugs to older people

When administering medications to older people, nurses can help to reduce the incidence of adverse drug reactions by:

- helping the older person to keep his or her mouth healthy;
- positioning the person upright;
- ensuring that the medication can be swallowed easily (e.g. elixirs can be used, tablets can be crushed but capsules should not be emptied. This is because the gelatin capsule ensures that the contents survive gastric acid and reach their appropriate place of absorption lower down the gastrointestinal tract.);
- encouraging the person to drink a full glass of liquid after taking the medicine;
- administering before or after food as appropriate for each drug;
- maintaining a normal fluid intake;
- helping prevent constipation;
- monitoring for signs of liver impairment;
- preventing urinary retention, monitoring for signs of renal impairment;
- questioning dosages, particularly for people with hepatic or renal impairment; and
- administering injections or topical applications carefully and observing for skin damage or bleeding.

Observing for drug-related problems

Nurses who are vigilant can often recognise when there are problems, and prevent these occurring, particularly when they know the older person well and recognise that something is wrong.

Adverse drug reactions can manifest in a wide variety of ways, but often within one of the 'Four I's' (previously known as the giants of geriatrics). There are mental instability, physical instability, incontinence, and immobility.

Mental instability, acute/toxic confusional state, or delirium, results because the older person has reduced functional reserve, and an adverse drug reaction may tip the balance so that the person can no longer maintain physiological equilibrium.

Physical instability or falls often occur because the drugs have impaired the person's postural control mechanisms and reduced the efficiency of the blood flow to the brain.

Incontinence can arise because a drug may increase the frequency of the desire to urinate, interfere with bladder or sphincter control, or impair the person's ability to respond quickly, for example by reducing mobility.

Immobility may result from the sedative effects of medications, or because the toxic effects leave the older person feeling weak.

In addition to observing for adverse drug reactions, nurses in care homes should also ensure that their own practice does not cause unnecessary problems for a resident. For example, many older people have taken sleeping tablets for years. On moving into a care home this habit continues. Some residents have even been awakened to be given their sleeping pill. Mainly because of the time the tablet is taken, there can be a reversal in sleep pattern. The client is then asleep all day and awake most of the night. There are many factors which contribute to insomnia besides night-time reliance on sedatives. Barbiturates are often considered as addictive. Temazepam is a popular drug used in nursing homes. It is also easily eliminated. If the problem of insomnia and the problems that may occur due to drugs taken, are discussed with the client, this is sometimes successful, and clients may prefer then to try an alternative, e.g. a hot drink instead of the pills.

Self-medication in care homes

The UKCC (1992c) has stated its support for the development of self-administration of medicines in nursing homes, wherever it is appropriate, and the necessary security and storage arrangements are available (paragraph 19).

Ideally when an older person moves into a care home, he or she retains responsibility for medicines, with support from nursing staff as necessary but, if a person is very physically or mentally frail, this may not be possible.

The advantages of self-medication are that it can boost morale by the person feeling in control and independent. The residents in most homes are able to understand why the drugs are prescribed and for what side-effects to observe. Those who administer their own medicines should be provided with a lockable cabinet or drawer. This can be time-consuming for carers if residents are unable to operate the locks. A record of drugs given to the resident should be kept.

Disadvantages include drug errors, particularly if the person is prone to memory lapse or losing the tablets, if there is difficulty removing child-proof lids or opening bobble packs, or if the tablets are small and the person has visual impairment.

Education is important, and the nurse should ensure that the older person understands when to take the medicines, how to take them, and any special precautions.

The responsibilities of the nurse

Registered nurses working in care homes should understand that it is their responsibility to ensure that safe practices in the administration of drugs are adhered to. This includes safe storage, the correct administration and disposal of drugs (UKCC, 1992c). The administration of drugs by one nurse only should be carried out in accordance with local policy. Unsafe practices can be missed if staff do not keep themselves updated on related topics. This may occur in nursing homes more than in a hospital setting because nursing home staff are often more isolated. In addition, many care home staff work part-time and some have only recently returned to work after several years' break (UKCC 1994b).

Each nurse is responsible for his or her actions, but the manager also has responsibility for ensuring that policies and procedures are in place, that all relevant information on standards of practice is obtained and communicated with others involved, and that teaching sessions are set up on a regular basis with staff attending these. (See Chapter 8: Management Matters.)

The UKCC Code of Professional Conduct states that a registered nurse should act always in a way as to promote and safeguard the well-being of the patient/client (UKCC 1992a).

Precautions

The policy of the nursing home regarding medications should be formulated in conjunction with the care team and the manager. This policy should be available for the registration officer on inspection of the home. It should include information regarding the ordering of drugs, storage, and safe and effective administration.

Supply of drugs

Drugs should be given when prescribed by the resident's general practitioner and dispensed by the community pharmacist. These should be reviewed on a monthly basis. A drug can be defined as 'any substance used in the diagnosis, treatment, cure, relief, or prevention of disease' (Webster, 1995). Any substances to be taken by a patient, even 'homely remedies', should be discussed and agreed with the person's doctor.

A record of drugs received and administered by the home must be maintained at all times. The pharmacists are advised of any changes in dosage in order for any changes in medication or labelling to be made.

Individual resident prescription charts are available and these should be signed and dated.

Storage and handling

Receipt of medications should be arranged so that safety and security are given adequate consideration. A record of drugs received and administered by the home should be maintained.

The medications should be stored in a locked cupboard or in the resident's own room. Medicines for external use, for example disinfectants, creams, items for treatment of pressure ulcers and blood testing reagents should be stored separately from medicines for internal use.

Eye drops, insulin and other medications for refrigeration should be stored in a drug refrigerator, according to the manufacturers' instructions.

Medicines should be stored in the containers in which they were dispensed. Medication containers should be removed following the completion of a supply. Any remaining medication should be returned to the pharmacy.

Controlled drugs should be stored centrally in a locked cupboard within a locked cupboard which is fixed to the wall. A controlled drug register should be kept in the home and controlled drugs should be given by a first-level nurse and checked by another person, for example, a second-level or student nurse.

Administration of drugs

Nurses who are responsible for the administration of drugs should be aware of the hazards due to the undesirable side-effects of drugs, particularly with multiple pathology and multiple prescribing. Several problems can arise for the nurse. She or he should be aware of the side-effects of each drug and be sufficiently observant to recognise them immediately.

New drugs are appearing on the market frequently but these drugs have been carefully tested. Unfortunately older people are not represented in these trials as significantly as they should be, particularly in terms of their proportion in the community of people who receive drugs.

Staff must be appropriately trained. Many second-level nurses have attended study days on drug administration and have been assessed as competent. They assume the responsibilities of a first-level nurse in this respect. In residential care home settings, either social workers or senior care assistants may administer drugs.

Medications should be administered in accordance with the doctor's instructions, and should be used for the resident for whom they have been prescribed, not for another resident. At the time of administration, the medication should be recorded and signed for.

In some care homes, medications arrive from the pharmacist in multiple dose packs, individually prepared for each resident.

The role of the general practitioner

The GP is responsible for the medical care of the residents in the home, but most decisions are made in conjunction with the nursing team. The GP should be consulted for advice, should contribute to the teaching of nurses, and should be considered as a member of the staff of the home. He or she should also review the drugs on a monthly basis in order to consider whether the resident should continue to take them.

The role of the pharmacist

The pharmacist has a valuable role. He or she provides information regarding various drugs, dispenses the drugs and can be active in teaching sessions to help nurses understand the different aspects of drug therapy. He or she may discuss difficulties and answer any questions.

Conclusion

Nurses in care homes have a vital role in helping residents to achieve health and well-being, but the multiple and complex changes which accompany ageing can be challenging. This chapter reviews some of the common symptoms experienced by older people, and refers to other chapters where more details can be found. Ideas for symptom relief and supportive activities have been offered. The chapter details the role and responsibilities of qualified nurses when using complementary, supplementary or alternative therapies, and when administering medications. Finally, the chapter emphasises that if a home offers consultation, choice, flexibility, meaningful activity, laughter and a positive environment, this can considerably help to overcome some of the challenging symptoms of ageing, and achieve greater health, well-being and quality of life for the older people who live in the home.

Useful contacts

British Complementary Medicine Association, St Charles Hospital, Exmoor Street, London W10 6DX.
Council for Complementary & Alternative Medicine, 179 Gloucester Place, London NW1 6DX.
Institute for Complementary Medicine, PO Box 194, London SE16 1QZ.

Aromatherapy
Aromatherapy Organisations Council, 3 Latymer Close, Braybrooke, Market Harborough, Leicester LE16 8LN.
International Federation of Aromatherapists, c/o Department of Continuing Education, The Royal Masonic Hospital, London W6 0TN.
International Society of Professional Aromatherapists, 41 Leicester Road, Hinckley, Leicester LE10 1LW.

Reflexology
The British Reflexology Association, 12 Pond Road, London SE3 9JL.

Therapeutic massage
The British Massage Therapy Council, c/o 9 Elm Road, Worthing, West Sussex.

Therapeutic touch
The Didsbury Trust, Sherbourne Cottage, Litton, Nr Bath, Somerset BA3 4PS.

References

Comfort, A. (1982) Sexuality in Later Life, in J.E. Birren and R.B. Shane (eds.) *Handbook of Mental Health and Ageing*. Englewood Cliffs, NJ: Prentice-Hall Inc.

Cooke, M. (1995) Complementary Therapies. In H.B.M. Heath (ed.) *Foundations in Nursing Theory and Practice.* London: Mosby

Counsel and Care (1991) No Such Private Places: A study of privacy and lack of privacy for residents in private and voluntary residential care and nursing homes in Greater London. London: Counsel and Care.

Dugan, D.O. (1989) Laughter and tears: best medicine for stress. *Nurse Forum,* **24**(1), 18.

Ebersole, P. and Hess, P. (1991) *Toward Healthy Aging: Human Needs and Nursing Reponse.* St Louis: Mosby.

Falk, G. and Falk, U. (1980) Sexuality and the Aged. *Nursing Outlook,* January 1980, 51–55.

Fulder, S. (1989) *The Handbook of Complementary Medicine.* London: Hodder and Stoughton.

Herr, K.A. and Mobily, P.R. (1994) Complexities of pain assessment in the eldery. *Journal of Gerontological Nursing,* **17**(4), 12.

Hill, L. and Oliver, N. (1993) Therapeutic Touch and Theory-based Mental Health Nursing. *Journal Psychosocial Nursing,* **31**(2), 19.

Kellett, J. (1989) Sex and the elderly. *Geriatric Medicine,* **19**(10), 17.

McCaffery, M. and Beebe, A. (1994) Pain in the elderly: special considerations. In M. McCaffery, A. Beebe and Latham J. (eds.) *Pain: Clinical manual for nursing practice.* London: Mosby.

Rankin-Box, D. (1992) European Developments in Complementary Medicine. *British Journal of Nursing,* **1**(2), 103.

Riley, A. (1994) Ageing and the physiology of sex. *Care of the Elderly,* March 1994, 92–96.

Sanderson, H. and Carter, A. (1994) Healing Hands. *Nursing Times,* **90** (11), 46.

Sayre-Adams, J. (1993) Therapeutic Touch – Principles and Practice. *Complementary Therapies Med,* **1**(2), 96.

Sayre-Adams, J. (1994) Therapeutic Touch: A Nursing Function. *Nursing Standard,* **8**.

Schultz, R. (1982) Emotionality and ageing: a theoretical and empirical analysis. *Journal of Gerontology,* **37**(1).

Sullivan, J.L. and Deane, D.M. (1988) Humour and health. *Journal of Gerontological Nursing,* **14**(1), 20.

Taylor, A.G. (1983) How effective is TENS for acute pain? *American Journal of Nursing,* **83**, 1171.

Trevelyan, J. and Booth, B., (1994) *Complementary Medicine for Nurses, Midwives and Health Visitors.* London: Macmillan.

United Kingdom Central Council for Nursing, Midwifery and Health Visiting (1994a) Register, No. 15. Autumn 1994. London: UKCC.

United Kingdom Central Council for Nursing, Midwifery and Health Visiting (1994b) Professional Conduct – Occasional Report on Standards of Nursing in Nursing Homes. London: UKCC.

United Kingdom Central Council for Nursing, Midwifery and Health Visiting (1992a) Code of Professional Conduct, London: UKCC.

United Kingdom Central Council for Nursing, Midwifery and Health Visiting (1992b) Scope of Professional Practice. London: UKCC.

United Kingdom Central Council for Nursing, Midwifery and Health Visiting (1992c) Standards for the Administration of Medicines. London: UKCC.

Walding, M.F. (1991) Pain, anxiety and powerlessness. *Journal of Advanced Nursing*, **16**, 388.

Webster, C. (1995) Administering Medication. In H.B.M. Heath (ed.) *Foundations in Nursing Theory and Practice*. London: Mosby.

White, C.B. (1982) Interests, Attitudes, Knowledge and Sexual History in relation to sexual behaviour in the instituionalised aged. *Archives of Sexual Beahviour*, **11**, 1, 11–21.

White, I. (1995) Controlling Pain. In Heath H.B.M. (ed.) *Foundations in Nursing Theory and Practice*. London: Mosby.

Williams, H. (1986) Humour and Healing: therapeutic effects in geriatrics. *Gerontologist*, **1**(3), 14.

Conclusion

In the future, the characteristics of older people will change, as different generations enter that section of society. Each generation will bring its own experiences and values. and distinct health and social care needs. Nurses will continue to face challenges and changes to the way they practice. All nurses who work with older people on a continuing basis need to demonstrate their value in this increasingly cost-efficiency-driven health and social care scenario.

The challenge is for nurses, both individually and collectively, to respond constructively in the face of potentially adverse conditions. While organisations and research units have the resources to undertake formalised studies, it is the individual nurse who provides the evidence which influences such studies. It is the responsibility of the individual nurse to develop his or her knowledge-base, communication and assertion skills, thus ensuring that older people's rights to nursing care are safeguarded.

By writing this book, individual nurses practising in a variety of settings have demonstrated their commitment to older people and to the nurses who work with them. The reader has much to contribute both in terms of sharing good practice, and reporting areas of concern.

In order to survive, nurses need to be continually challenging the way in which they work, and developing new ways of working. Nurse practitioner roles hold exciting opportunities, and demographic trends indicate that nurses who are highly skilled in the care of older people will be in considerable demand in the future.

The key to good practice is that the older person's rights, needs and choices will remain at the centre of the care. Older people, no matter how physically or mentally vulnerable, should be able to express and act upon their wants and needs and should be helped, where necessary, both to express and act upon their choices.

A key challenge will be the continuing resistance of the assumption that it is the high-technology care that needs the most highly-skilled nurses. We hope that this book demonstrates the immense skill required for high-touch rather than high-tech care, and the enormous potential for nurses committed to working with older people.

Index